**This book**
tells you how you can prevent the lessening of physical
capacities we all fear that sets in around 40 and what you
have to do to be physically and psychologically fit during
your 50's and 60's. Physical exercise is the answer: Dr.
Walter Noder has presented the successful program of the
Bad Salzuflen Exercise School in a form that enables
everyone to practice heart circulation training (HCT)—in
correct doses—for himself. And that means: remaining at an
optimal level of fitness and alertness both on the job and in
leisure time.

**Walter Noder, M.D.**
Specialist in Internal Medicine, Dr. Walter Noder was born
in Ludwigshafen/Rhein in 1926. He studied medicine and
psychology in Würzburg and Heidelberg and received his
doctorate and *venia legendi* in Internal Medicine in Münster
in 1967. Dr. Noder was head of the Institute for Preventive
Medicine and Psychotherapeutic Rehabilitation at the
University of Münster and managing physician of the
Exercise Center at Staatsbad Salzuflen until 1974. He is
currently chief physician of the Rhein-Lahn Clinic in
Lahnstein.

# Speaking of:
# Fitness Over 40

# The
# Medical
# Adviser Series

Medical
Adviser
Series

Walter Noder, M.D.

# Speaking of:
# Fitness Over 40

Keeping Active and Healthy
Through Improved Circulation

translated by: Susan Ray, Ph.D.

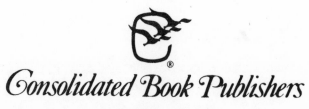

*Consolidated Book Publishers*

NEW YORK • CHICAGO

Library of Congress Catalog Card Number: 78-72872
ISBN: 0-8326-2236-2

Originally published in German under the title Leistungsfähig
über 40, copyright © 1978 by Gräfe und Unzer Verlag, München.

# Contents

# It's up to You

For most people the age of forty marks the zenith of their performance and experiential capacities. "From then on it's all downhill" runs the refrain, and some, looking back, will have to admit that this, unfortunately, is also true in their own case.

But it does not have to be. It's up to us to extend our period of optimal productivity and experience and to remain 40 years old for ten or perhaps even 20 years.

Yet, this is only half the story: heart attacks among people under forty are surprisingly numerous. One adult in three has a major or minor cardiac circulatory ailment. Especially affected by this are the men and women in managerial positions for whom the problem of "fitness over forty" frequently decides the success or failure of a career. Today we know that proper amounts of physical exercise have restorative effects on an impaired circulation. Even among people with a risk of heart attack, cardiac exercise, when properly administered, pays off.

I have been repeatedly asked by people who have felt the positive effects of physical training within the context of an active cure at Bad Salzuflen—frequently for the first time in their lives—as to how they should design their exercise program once they return home. This book gives the answer. It presents the successful program of the Exercise

School at Bad Salzuflen in a format that enables everyone to set up his own cardiac circulation training program at home. In addition, it contains advice and help for everyone who wants to remain fit and healthy and who is also prepared to do something—namely the right thing—to attain this goal.

This book is the product of years of practical experience in dealing with the problems of people who have actually been able to redirect their will toward the improvement of the physical capacity of their bodies. It contains the findings of my own scientific research in the field of functional analysis of the cardio-pulmonary system (the heart-lung circulatory system), and is the result of long and often painstaking practical efforts in making the findings of sports medicine and preventive health care available even to those who, as adults, are looking for some physical activity for the first time and who are unable to avail themselves of the expert advice of a teacher or physician well-versed in sports.

I would also like to say what this book is not: it is neither a textbook for sports nor a sports manual, and definitely not a textbook on the treatment of functional disabilities. In no case is it a guide for the sick. For them, the one and only source of competent advice is their own physician.

At this point I should like to thank all those people whose knowledge and experience have consciously or unconsciously gone into the making of this book. To list them here individually or even to weigh their contributions would be impossible. Instead, I should like to name only three as representative of many: Professor M. Hochrein, my highly respected first clinical instructor; Dr. K. V. Baum, my long-time friend and fellow combatant, the first successful physician-director of the Exercise Center at Bad Salzuflen; and Dr. A. Drews, my esteemed colleague.

I should also like to thank the publisher and staff of Gräfe-und-Unzer-Verlag in Munich for their incentive and assistance in putting this book together.

*Walter Noder, M.D.*

# 1. Remaining 40 for 20 Years

My readers will have bought this book because they are beginning to notice that the conditions determining their lives call for a significant extension of their phase of full intellectual and physical fitness. Also, the multiplicity of their potential experiences makes it desirable to maintain this phase of optimal vitality for as long as possible. Miracles are rare in our times—but not because there is a lack of those phenomena that one might describe as such, but because we have learned that every effect must have its cause—even if we are unable to recognize it immediately. We have learned to explain, that is to rationalize, the many "wonders" that do surround us.

*A realizable miracle?*

Remaining 40 for 20 years would be one such miracle. We all know that no one is capable of stopping time, let alone of determining when and how long it should stand still. Obviously, we all grow older with every passing year. Yet no one judges a person's appearance according to his or her age, but rather according to how the person looks, behaves, thinks—in short, according to his or her overall manner of handling the years. We all know older people who appear youthful and younger people who appear older than they are. Even so, it is not an exactly common occurrence that a 60-year-old is taken for 40 or vice versa.

Yet, we can see from this that there must be

11

circumstances that accelerate or retard a person's biological aging process, even though the natural course of time is equally binding for us all. If such circumstances do exist, it must also be possible to discover them—perhaps not all, but surely the most important ones—and to alter them, as far as is possible, to conform to our desires; in other words, to force the "biological clock" to slow down. When seen in this light, the promise of being able to remain 40 for 20 years—if you do not take it too literally—is surely no pipe-dream, and to a great extent it is in your power to make this "miracle" come true.

*Slowing down the biological clock*

Every change in a person's condition or course of life presupposes abilities or energies that can effect these changes. Obviously, this applies to the speeding up or slowing down of a mechanical clock, but it is equally true of the course of our own biological clock, the aging process. In other words, we have to invest energy, do something, if we want to retard the aging process.

This book will help you do just that. I should like to give you several facts that are meant to help you to decide
● what you can do
● how you will have to start, and
● why you have to do exactly *this*—and in a very definite way—and not something else in order to extend your period of optimal physical fitness and maximum experiential capacity.

You have to do it yourself. No one has yet amassed a fortune by merely studying and not practicing the laws of economics.

Nevertheless, no one will engage in such activity, take the trouble to spend energy and invest time and even money if it does not fulfill two requirements:
a) The desired goal has to promise increased happiness. I consider this requirement already fulfilled, for otherwise you would never have so much as looked at this book.
b) You must be convinced that the program suggested represents the best way to attain this goal.

This presupposes a basic understanding of certain

12

biological processes. A little theory is also unavoidable. I shall therefore present several important facts allegorically by using examples from daily life.

# The Physical Slowdown at 40—Why?

The human body is an extremely complicated organism consisting of an inconceivably large number of microscopic building blocks called cells. Basically, these cells are individual independent living organisms with their own energy supply (metabolism), and this makes them individually viable in a suitable environment. They are merged into cellular units (tissues) within the body, and different types of tissues (muscle, nerve, or glandular cell tissues, for example) unite cells of the same shape and function. Specific tissue types with "productive functions" are combined with other tissue types that fulfill predominantly "auxiliary functions" to form organs (kidneys, lungs, stomach, etc.).

*The organism, its construction and function*

Individual organs that work toward the same end constitute organ systems, such as the nervous system, the digestive system, etc., and the combination of these, in turn, distinguishes one organism from another. The organizational structure, the division of labor, and the differentiation we can see in this suggest comparison with a state. The latter, too, is composed of many discrete individuals whose autonomy is kept in check by other individuals. On the other hand, it is they who are responsible for the existence of these autonomous individuals in the first place through their specialization, differentiation, division of labor, and cooperation. In both cases we find units, organizations, and even certain hierarchical structures with steering mechanisms that characterize the symbiosis of many discrete individuals in a highly organized community. Thus, just as a state needs a long period of time to alter its external form

13

and its functions (we are disregarding exceptional situations here), while its citizens continue to change, so is our body, too, no longer absolutely identical with what it was yesterday. This is blatantly perceptible to everyone during the period of growth and development, and is also readily discernible in one's changing outward appearance. Yet, this process does not stop in adulthood by any means. Cells are constantly dying and new ones are constantly being formed.

This permanent state of change in our bodies, which we do not directly perceive ourselves, is the prerequisite for those structural changes that we call development and aging, as well as the prerequisite for the organism's ability to adapt to changing external or internal conditions.

*The aging process*

In order to understand how this aging process takes place, we have to look at the process of cellular regeneration in more detail. We know that, as a result of the phenomena of wear, the cells of our body have only a limited life span and therefore have to be constantly replaced by new cells. In order to do this, every cell carries within it its own blueprint of shape and function in the form of a code and is thus able to duplicate itself upon a certain signal. (This generalized explanation has certain exceptions that have no bearing on our context but which in principle do limit the theoretical life expectancy of an individual). In the course of a lifetime this process of duplication is repeated very frequently at intervals that differ in keeping with the individual cell type. This procedure can be compared to photocopying a letter. Each new copy is a copy of the preceding one. The copies become poorer and poorer in quality, until, after a number of reproductions, the text has become almost illegible.

*Reproduction of the cells with a decline in quality*

We can imagine that the cells of our bodies are constantly changing in much the same way during the course of a long life and many reproductions. Yet, the changes in their shape are less striking than those in their essentially more important function: they are becoming older and with that the functional indicators of the whole organism are necessarily changing. This aging process applies in principle

14

to every series of cellular reproduction starting with the first day of a person's development.

Strictly speaking, therefore, we start aging biologically from the moment our body first begins to develop out of the union of our mother's egg with our father's sperm. According to this, then, our "productive capacity" and the intensity of our "feeling for life" would actually have to steadily decrease from the moment of conception.

*Productive capacity and feeling for life*

There are essentially two reasons why this is not the case: a person's so-called productive capacity is dependent not only upon the quality, but also upon the quantity, and therefore the volume, of the cell functions. During the first decades of life, the quantity increases more than the quality decreases. In addition, the "operational curves" differ: they reach their zenith at different times. Thus, the curve of the growth functions is already again approaching the zero point when the curve of sexual potency is reaching its climax and the curve of intellectual functions is entering the range of its sharpest ascent.

Productive capacity and vitality are not absolute quantities, but are relative as far as environmental conditions or requirements are concerned. Under the conditions that determine our lives, intellectual functions, such as knowledge and experience, have a higher priority than bodily functions. Yet, the intellectual functions—as we have said—reach their highest capacity considerably later than the physical functions do. As long as the "resultant"* of all functions is increasing, we feel fit and strong, our feeling for life is "pleasurable." If this trend becomes negative, we perceive it as a "slowdown," our feeling for life becomes unpleasurable. Our creative power, our ability to enjoy and our *joie de vivre* diminish. For many people, this state of affairs sets in around the age of 40 because it is at this point in time that the bodily functions have already

---

* This term comes from physics and describes the direction and size of the action of several vector forces, themselves differing with regard to direction and size, which act on a center of mass (a parallelogram of forces, for example).

15

clearly passed their zenith and the intellectual functions are no longer increasing sharply enough to keep the overall trend positive—the psychological aging process is beginning.

*The search for compensa- tory gratification*

The unconscious striving toward a compensatory gratification now results in a search for sources of substitute pleasures, primarily those relating to food. They are easy to develop, promise a quick attainment of the desired result, and can be relied upon to repeat it.

Oral gratification, to mention just one example, tested, proven, and recommended in critical situations ever since time immemorial, gains in importance and frequently becomes a constantly obliging, but false, friend. So much has already been said and written in recent times about the consequences of food that is too rich or, more importantly, does not meet our nutritional needs, that I need only refer my readers to the pertinent literature. Overweight alone would be the least deleterious of these consequences.

The search for these substitute pleasures almost always results in a clear and speedy impairment of many bodily functions, frequently even in genuine illnesses and thus always in an additional disturbance of one's well-being. The unconsciously sought compensatory gratification is not attained; instead, a fatal carousel of negative, mutually reinforcing effects is set in motion.

It is up to us, then to break out of this vicious circle, or, better yet, not to let it start in the first place.


# Is There a Fountain of Youth?

How can we prevent or temporarily protract this slowdown of our physical capacities, decelerate this drop in productivity and thus maintain an optimistic and pleasurable state of health?

We have seen that the tone of our feeling for life is determined by the restraining effect of the "resultants" upon all physical and intellectual functions. Many, indeed most of

16

these functions are subject to a consistent periodic course which we are not able to influence, or rather, not yet. Still, this does not apply to all functions. One of the bodily functions essential for good health—namely, our capacity of physical productivity—can be especially and effectively influenced by exercise or training. This last remark borders on a truism, and yet, here we have a general biological law in a particularly impressive formula: functions that are practiced can be improved; functions that are not practiced deteriorate.

*Functions that are practiced can be improved*

If a person succeeds in maintaining his or her physical capacities, or in slowing down the natural, age-conditioned involution process—the process of regeneration—or if he or she succeeds in improving his or her physical productive capabilities, then not only will the other bodily functions be likewise positively affected, but so will the "resultants" that determine our state of health and which derive from all these functions. The physical slowdown is diminished and temporarily protracted and the course of the biological clock is thus decelerated.

Prolonging one's period of optimal physical and experiential capacity, or, in other words, remaining 40 for 20 years, thus becomes a real possibility.

Up until now I have spoken in very general terms about the "capacity of physical productivity" as if it were a clearly defined term. This, however, is by no means the case, for there are many different physical capabilities. Let's imagine a gymnast, a weight lifter, and a marathon runner, to mention only three examples. Each of these disciplines requires a great capacity of physical productivity, though obviously of a very differing kind. For gymnastics, agility and "body control," the so-called neuromuscular coordination, has to be especially and highly developed. In the case of a weight lifter or a marathon runner, on the other hand, these abilities are of lesser importance. For a weight lifter, absolute muscle strength plays the major role, whereas the marathon runner must possess endurance above all else.

17

Absolute strength, general aerobic* endurance and
neuromuscular coordination are the three most important
components of a physical productive capacity. Of course,
they are essential for all athletic exercises, but, as we have
seen, their importance varies for the different disciplines.
The question thus arises as to which of these components of
the physical capacity plays the decisive role in good health?
Are the different components equivalent in their effect, and
if not, why not?

We will try to answer this question with an example
drawn from a very familiar aspect of daily life, the
automobile. Imagine two trucks, which we will call "A" and
"B". "A" is a heavy vehicle with a strong body, a high
maximum load (strength), and four wheel drive (agility and
coordination), but with a relatively weak motor (endurance).
"B" is a light vehicle with the usual turning radius, but
with a very powerful motor. Both vehicles should travel at
an average speed of 60mph.

Based on these features, everyone will picture "A" as a
"slow crate" and "B" as a "hot rod". Everyone will feel
that 60mph will prove to be a problem for "A" over the
long run because it has to be driven constantly at the limit
of its productive capacity, because it will "run out of steam"
on inclines, and because it will only be able to pass other
vehicles under certain conditions. These problems will surely
not present themselves in "B's" case—it can perform these
feats "blindfolded."

If a car had feelings, "B" would surely feel better than
"A", for we know from personal experience that good
health is a direct function of reserve capacities. Whenever
we approach the limit of our physical abilities, in any field,
we perceive it as exertion and as "unpleasurable."

Now, what is true for the motor of a car is true for the
heart of a human being. Our heart is the organ that is

---

* from the Greek word *aer* meaning air. It denotes the field of
physical productivity in which the amount of oxygen necessary for
the production of energy is fully available.

responsible for whether or not the cells of our body can be sufficiently supplied with building materials or fuel under all conditions of stress and with the oxygen that is so important for energy output.

*Our heart, the "achilles heel" of the body*

If I may be forgiven a mixed metaphor, the heart is, as it were, the achilles heel of our body. Its failure causes immediate and extreme consequences, whereas disturbances of the other organs, at least for a certain period, can be counterbalanced to a large extent.

The body is as physically fit as its heart, a person is as young as his circulatory system, and it is no accident that the concepts of "old" and "hardened" (in the sense of degenerative changes in bodily vessels) are used almost synonymously. Regardless of how impressive a person's muscles are or whether or not he can scratch his right ear with his left foot—if his circulatory system and primarily his heart are weak, then "it's all over."

So the question as to which one of the components of our physical productive capacity plays the major role almost answers itself. A continuous aerobic productive capacity and cardiac fitness are just about identical; of all the components of this capacity, the greatest significance as far as good health is concerned accrues to overall aerobic endurance, continuous productive capacity, or to "stamina."

*Summary*

In summary:
1) In order to prolong the period of optimal physical and experiential capacity, we must prevent the physical slowdown.
2) We can lessen and temporarily protract the slowdown if we manage to maintain our capacity of physical productivity.
3) The essential component of this physical ability is endurance.
4) The only way to improve or maintain one's endurance is to train.

# 2. Training

## What You Should Know about Training

*In this book, the term* training *is used to mean the regular systematic repetition of definite exercises aimed at increasing a person's physical capacity.*

As mentioned above, in keeping with a biological law, the functions that are practiced improve. Those functions that are not practiced, on the other hand, deteriorate. For those organs that have to perform these functions, then, this means that as far as their construction, their size, and their supply and excretory systems are concerned, they are geared to a certain function that is required of them under *normal* circumstances. This process is comparable to a factory whose productive capacity in the long term is also geared to demand. If the demand increases more than the short term, then the existing equipment is charged beyond its critical limits. In-plant bottlenecks in production occur and they in turn trigger measures that result in an overall increase of the productive capacity.

*Training—measured doses of overexertion*

The biological term for this process is "training." It is a proportionately measured overexertion of specific organs with the purpose of "increasing productive capacity", of

21

increasing one's fitness.

In light of the different components of physical fitness, you have already discovered that training obviously produces different effects. Accordingly, there are also various forms, types, and methods of training that are appropriate for the respective goal. Proper preparation is crucial for the success or failure of any undertaking, and this applies to physical training as well.

*This is why I now want to explain:*
- *how often, how long, how intensively, and*
- *when you ought to train;*
- *how you can best go about your training;*
- *what clothing you should choose, and*
- *what rules apply regarding your way of life, your diet, and your use of stimulants.*

Following that I want to discuss several safety rules, for the purpose of our efforts is to improve our state of health, not to impair it.

A training program designed to increase our physical capacities will concentrate primarily upon two organ systems:
- the support system (bones, muscles, tendons, ligaments, and joints) as well as
- the oxygenation system, consisting of the lungs on the one hand and of the heart and blood vessels on the other.

In a later chapter entitled "Basic Knowledge" I shall delve more deeply into these matters. Here I should just like to say that the more endurance components a training program contains, the greater will be the stress exerted upon the oxygenation system and thus on the heart. But, any training program, even if properly administered, involves a certain amount of "overexertion," and it is important to understand the risks this involves. The extent of this risk varies according to the individual and the activity; moreover, it can be controlled, and above all, minimized (that is, the risk can be kept as small as possible). We shall return to this point at the end of the chapter.

*We have to be able to recognize the indications that tell us when a "stress" or "measured overexertion" has reached the point where it can provide a positive training effect. This is very important.*

# The Prerequisites

*Constant training stimulants*

In principle, the innumerable movements we make every day represent a training stimulant. Without these permanent stimulants our support system would atrophy. In order to increase the heart's capacity for continuous production, it is not necessary to do heavy physical work all day. This exertion would be impractical and the result fatigue, but not good health.

● *All one need do is trigger a brief, but concentrated training stimulant at regular intervals.*
● *This training stimulant has to increase in strength in indirect proportion to the intensity of the effect and in direct proportion to the length of time between two successive stimulants.*
● *If the duration of the stimulant is too short, no effect is produced; if the pauses between the stimulants are too long, the first stimulant has already died away before the second one sets in.*

*Findings of sports medicine and preventive health care*

Sports medicine and preventive health care have been working on this problem for the last few decades and have obtained a number of results that can be briefly summarized as follows:
● In order to increase the absolute strength of a muscle, it is enough to strain this muscle to its maximum strength at

23

least once a day for 8 seconds at a time. The more frequently one does this, the greater the increase in strength. There is no benefit worth mentioning in prolonging the duration of this tension.

● This kind of training—which is called isometric training—does not lead to an improvement in the fitness of the oxygenation system and thus also not to an increase in aerobic endurance, but merely to muscle growth and an increase of its absolute strength.

*Exercises aimed at improving aerobic endurance and thus the oxygenation capacity have to fulfill five requirements:*
*1) They have to be the right kind of exercises, that is, they must be dynamic, they have to involve movement.*
*2) At least 1/6 of all the body's muscles must be exercised at the same time.*
*3) The intensity of the exercise has to be high enough that the pulse rate per minute produced by it is raised about 60% of its starting rate. A person should reach a minimum rate of 170 minus his/her age, but should not exceed a rate of 220 minus his/her own age.*
*4) The exercises have to be maintained at this intensity for at least 6 minutes without interruption and must*
*5) be performed at least 4 times a week on different days, and the pauses between the exercises may not exceed 2 days.*

Prolonging the exercise periods increases their efficacy.

To maintain a once attained greater degree of fitness, an exercise program of twice a week is enough, provided that the length of the period is not less than 30 minutes each.

In light of the criteria specified above, a great number, indeed most, athletic activities are eliminated right from the start if the goal is an improvement of aerobic endurance.

Only the following activities remain:
- Mountain hiking or brisk walking on level ground
- running (jogging)
- cycling
- rowing or paddling
- swimming
- conditioning calisthenics.

I shall go into these points in more detail in the chapter on "Training Programs."

# Training As an Integral Part of the Daily Routine

The exact time of day that proves most expedient for training can only be determined on the basis of a person's individual habits and career obligations. Yet, we can make the following general statement:

*Early and late starters*

*so-called "early starters" train better in the morning before work, and "late starters" should schedule their training for the late afternoon.*

For most people the time directly after rising is inadvisable. An organism that is still attuned to rest should not be required to perform, for this greatly increases the danger of possible injury. The unavoidable exceptions to this only confirm the rule.

I myself follow this schedule: after rising I put on my track suit and do my morning exercises in the form of the basic calisthenics presented in this book.

I follow this with a shower, after which I am properly awake and fit for my professional work. I postpone my actual training program until the afternoon.

*The ideal schedule for training*

When I am free to allocate my time as I wish, as during vacations, for example, I keep to the following schedule which I should like to recommend to all those readers who

25

are also free to determine how their time is spent.

- Immediately after rising, a 10-minute morning exercise period including stretching, limbering up, tension, and breathing exercises according to the model of "basic calisthenics" (see p. 36)
- Then my morning toilette, including an unhurried hot and cold shower
- followed by a light breakfast consisting mainly of carbohydrates.
- Rest for 20 to 30 minutes and then a 10-minute walk.
- I now run through the woods for 20 minutes or do some other appropriate exercise that serves to improve endurance.
- Another shower (but this time avoiding cold water).
- An additional half hour of rest and then
- a hearty breakfast.

After this routine you will feel so much in shape that you will want to move mountains.

# Proper Clothing Is a Must

Now to the wardrobe. You will perhaps be grumbling: "It's all the same. It doesn't matter what I wear, the important thing is that I move." Actually, your clothing is essential, and if I now devote several pages to this topic, I do so for two reasons:

- because I know that many people, and mainly those who have not regularly participated in sports and who perhaps do not have an exactly ideal athletic figure, are reluctant to appear in public in sports clothes, and
- because inappropriate clothing increases the danger of accidents.

You may already have noticed during television broadcasts of sporting events that athletes seem to be preoccupied with taking off and putting on their track suits. They are not doing this to kill time but rather to keep their muscles warm.

26

Every athletic activity places a severe mechanical strain, primarily of a stretching nature, upon the muscles, and especially where the tendons begin.

*Since cold muscles are more tense and have a lower blood supply compared to well warmed muscles, they are not only less fit than warm ones, but they are also more susceptible to injury.*

However, I do not intend to talk about torn muscle fibers here. Since cold muscles have a reduced circulation, the metabolites produced during the strain are not only dramatically increased, but they also can not be completely removed. Therefore, they remain in the muscle and can cause a Charley horse.

In other words, what is true for top athletes in optimal condition should also be proper and fitting for us leisure time athletes. The motto, then, is "keep warm." Our clothing should let the air through as well as allow proper breathing so that no heat can accumulate, for there is a great increase in the conversion of energy in the working muscles during intensive physical activity. Heat (the so-called "combustion heat") is set free and has to be removed. Yet, at the same time care must be taken that the clothing can absorb the perspiration that is activated to regulate body heat.

*Keep warm is the motto*

Obviously, the outfit also has to be both light and comfortable in order not to hinder movement. Therefore, no one should hesitate to wear a track suit for every training session, even if he/she exercises at home, because that is what these suits are made for. If you do not have a track suit, a loose pair of trousers that do not hinder mobility and a sweater will do in the beginning. This outfit, though, is unsuitable for an endurance training such as running.

Lately we see increasing numbers of factory produced creations that seem more suited for a fashion show than for athletic activities. Let's not deceive ourselves. The appearance of the outfit is not the important consideration,

27

but how practical it is, and finally, we should keep in mind that a track suit has to be laundered now and then. So, if you are toying with the idea of getting a woolen track suit, remember that these outfits do not wash very well and that you can buy two suits of a cotton blend for the price of one woolen one.

*Cotton
underwear*

Underwear should be snug and flexible, and, if possible, made of pure cotton. Long underwear and a woolen undershirt can be added for outdoor exercises in the winter. The short pants and jersey outfit, typical of competitions, is unsuitable for training, as are the leotards sometimes preferred by women.

And now a word about shoes: practical shoes are absolutely essential for outdoor athletic activities, and especially for running. Both men and women should wear shoes of soft leather with a solid but flexible, flat sole and no heel. They must provide solid support for the foot, have to fit well and should have an innersole. The color and number of decorative stripes is totally irrelevant.

*First get
accustomed
to flat shoes*

In the beginning flat shoes can cause discomfort around the achilles tendon, especially for women who are accustomed to wearing only high-heeled shoes. For this reason women should get used to walking in flat shoes for a while and, if need be, stretch their calf muscles with the help of goal-oriented exercises before they start their training program (see goal-oriented calisthenics—Running, p. 86). In the event of serious trouble or for the transition period, heel cushions are very useful and can be purchased in shoe stores or orthopedic specialty shops.

# A Sensible Life-Style
# Makes Training Easier

*The effect and especially the success of a training program are greatly influenced by life-style and certain habits.*

It is not my intention to present you with a list of forbidden things or to encourage you to lead an ascetic life. But the least you should know is that nicotine, for example, clearly impairs the effect of training and why it does so. But before we go into this we want to discuss the factors of life-style and diet.

Surely all of you have heard or read that prior to a competition or during training top athletes follow a special schedule and avoid everything that can be described as "little sins." There is no question that proper nourishment is very important for health, fitness, and well-being. There is also no question that excesses of any kind, primarily when they lead to fatigue or nervous overstimulation, reduce one's efficiency. This is true not only for the top athletes, but for all of us, and especially prior to competitive or challenging situations.

In my view, such measures are predominantly a psychological problem. Top athletes want to win the competition. Yet, only one can win, and it is frequently the little mistakes that determine victory or defeat. Still, we can bear a defeat psychologically more easily if we are convinced that we have done everything and have omitted nothing that might contribute to success.

This occasionally results in the grotesque situation that out of a proper recognition of the detrimental effects of an excessive life-style, a person strives toward and even practices another equally harmful life-style.

Such considerations are of little importance for those people who do not want to engage in competitive sports.

*Therefore, you need change nothing in your life-style,*

*Proper*
*nourishment,*
*enough sleep*

*in your life habits, and in your diet*
- *if you get enough sleep*
- *if you observe moderation in all things*
- *if you watch your weight, that is, eat a proper diet.*
  *These rules apply to everybody.*

And now a word about nicotine. We all know that smoking is harmful or at least not conducive to good health. And surely we also know that nicotine is toxic to our vessels, impairs circulation, and that carbon monoxide is inhaled along with the smoke. This carbon monoxide "blocks" the red hemoglobin from absorbing oxygen. This

*Smoking*
*means less*
*oxygen*

means not only less oxygen, but also less energy producing nutritive materials and less building material for the cells of the organs that have to perform the work.

Even habitual smokers cannot deny that the effects of nicotine are detrimental and can even be dangerous for the heart and the muscles during periods of stress—even if the stress is properly administered. I do not wish to go into further details about the problem of smoking, since it is obvious to all that nicotine and physical activity or training do not mix well. With nicotine a person not only clearly impairs the results of his training, but he can also expose himself to considerable dangers.

*I should therefore like to strongly recommend that*
- *immediately before and*
- *immediately after strenuous physical activities you refrain absolutely from smoking.*

By "immediately before" I mean a period of at least 30 minutes and by "immediately after" I mean as long as it takes for the increased activity that was caused by the stress to readjust itself. It will be less difficult for you to follow this recommendation than you will perhaps at first think. The need to smoke reduces itself almost automatically soon after your training begins.

# Safety Rules

And now for a few safety rules. You will immediately ask: "Can I train without exposing myself to any danger and how much can I expect of myself?" The first part of the question is easy to answer. You may train if you are in good health and the activity does not result in any ailments. Your age makes no difference here.

*If it is possible, you may and should train even if you are no longer or not yet in a good state of health. However, only your physician can make this decision on an individual basis.*

*It can sometimes be difficult (at least for yourself) to judge whether or not you are healthy. If you have even the slightest doubt about this, no matter how old you are, you should immediately consult a physician. Obviously, while consulting your physician you should clearly express your intention of starting a physical training program and you should ask whether and what risks this might possibly pose for you.*

*When in doubt, consult a physician*

There is no magic age after which a person must necessarily consult a physician before he embarks on a training program nor is there one that marks the end of a person's relative immunity against the risks involved in starting an athletic activity. The beginning especially of chronic diseases is frequently not perceived by the person affected. Yet, these are the very illnesses that appear more frequently the older you get. Thus, as you get older it becomes more important that you consult a physician before starting a training program, even if you have previously participated in sports activities but have neglected your training for some time. It is therefore impossible to specify a certain age beyond which you have to consult a physician before you start to train; anything I might say could be the absolutely wrong thing for you.

31

All those people who have actively participated in sports ever since they were young do not face this problem. All the others, however, who as adults are first finding or rediscovering their way to physical activity should be "reinsured", as it were, by their physician.

*How much you may expect of yourself depends solely upon your present productive capacities. This establishes your limits quite automatically. If you are healthy, the concern that you might perhaps overburden your heart is unfounded.*

If you are not fully capable of bearing stress (or are limited in your physical abilities), your physician will tell you how you should proceed. A healthy heart, however, can bear more than you might think.

In the following pages I shall advise you repeatedly to proceed slowly with your training program. I do so less out of a concern for your heart than to protect you against injury. The bearer and mediator of any training program is your support system, in other words, your muscles, tendons, ligaments, joints, and bones. Every injury, even the so-called minor ones, either impair your training ability or cripple it completely. The many complications that interrupt training, even the physical therapy of heart patients, have nothing to do with the heart, but are of an orthopedic nature.

*Seven safety rules to avoid injuries*

*Make a mental note, therefore, of the following seven safety rules, and, most importantly, observe them:*
*1) Begin every exercise at a deliberately slow pace, not only when you begin to train, but later on as well. Only after you have warmed up can you go to full speed. After all, you wouldn't treat your automobile any differently.*
*2) Do not exercise on a full stomach.*
*3) Fatigue and physical exhaustion increase the danger of accidents.*

32

*4) If you feel sick or have a fever, you belong in bed and not on the playing field.*

*5) Discomforts during or after the training should urge you to consult a physician immediately. Only he can decide whether these discomforts are harmless or not.*

*6) Take care not to stop your training abruptly, but rather let the stress wind down slowly.*

*7) Do not take a cold shower after stress. The motto is "keep warm", even after training.*

# 3. Training Programs

Once you have decided to start your own training program in order to improve your heart circulation and thus your endurance capacity, there is a wide range of activities to choose from:

*Activities of the heart circulatory training program*

- *mountain hiking or brisk walking on even ground*
- *running (jogging)*
- *cycling*
- *rowing*
- *swimming*
- *conditioning calisthenics.*

These various activities have differing prerequisites that render some of these sports unsuitable for some people. However, I should like to start by illustrating an exercise program that
- can be performed by everyone (at their own individual pace)
- is practically without risk
- makes no demands as far as special equipment is concerned and therefore can be practiced everywhere—at home, on a trip, indoors or out.

35

# The Basic Exercises

The basic exercises are designed to put stress on the most important muscle groups in a certain sequence and to exercise the major joints. For this reason they are just as well suited for morning exercises directly after rising as for limbering up or warm-up exercises prior to an endurance training program. These exercises should become one of your daily habits and should be performed at the same time every day—the best time is in the morning right after getting up.

*Becoming a daily habit*

Laziness, lack of time, and other adverse circumstances will provide constant temptations to cancel a day's exercise. Resist this temptation! The longer you practice these

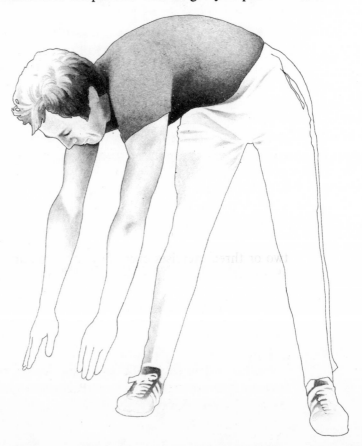

exercises, the more they will become a part of you, and after a while they will have become as natural as brushing your teeth.

● *Start the exercises slowly and only gradually increase the pace. This is particularly important for senior citizens.*
● *Do the exercises exactly as described, but do not try to force yourself. Certain exercises become easier with time. Training has to be strenuous, but it should never hurt.*

# Fit for Every Day

*Exercise out of doors or in front of open window*

The following pages contain 13 illustrated basic exercises that can be done in about ten minutes at a moderate pace*. You should begin with these if you have never been active in sports or if you have been inactive for any length of time. If possible, choose a spot near a window so that you can fill your lungs with fresh air while you exercise.

The charts at the end of the book are meant to measure your progress. In the beginning of your training you should record every day of completed exercises.

After two or three weeks you will feel ready to do more. At this point you should graduate to the exercises described in chapter 4. I recommend that you perform an additional two or three exercises every day until you are eventually able to do all 22 of them in one session.

---

\* You may obtain a poster of these basic exercises by writing to: Exercise Poster, Consolidated Book Publishers, 420 Lexington Avenue, New York, New York, 10017.

# Basic Exercises
# For Heart Circulatory Training

## 1 Warm Up

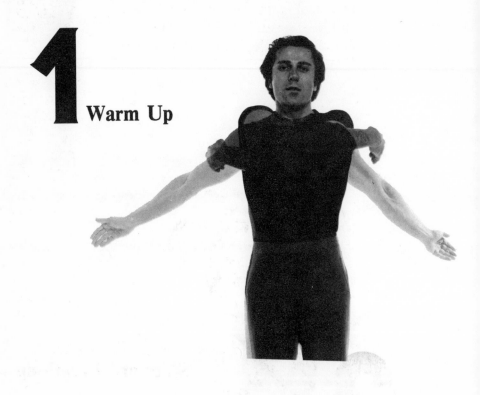

Arms stretched out sideways forming 45°
angle with body. Draw arms backward, then
forward vigorously, crossing them in front of
the chest, and following through to the back.
Repeat 10 to 15 times.

# 2 Stretching

Clasp hands in front of body and while tensing all muscles, inhale and raise hands directly in front of body and over head. Then relax the muscles while exhaling. Repeat 3 to 5 times.

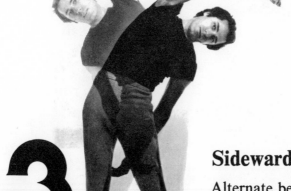

# 3 Sideward Breathing

Alternate between bending the body sideways to the left and then to the right. Breathe in and out to the rhythm of the bends, right in, left out, etc. Repeat 5 times each side.

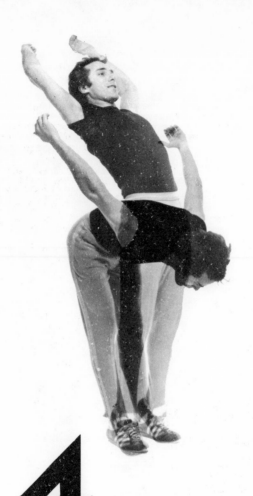

# **4** Forward Body Bend

With legs stretched, knees straight, and
upper body erect, bend from hips and,
while exhaling, swing arms vigorously
through, up, and behind your back.
Return to starting position via a deep
squat and inhale while standing up.
Repeat 10 to 15 times.

# 5 Arm Circles With Hops

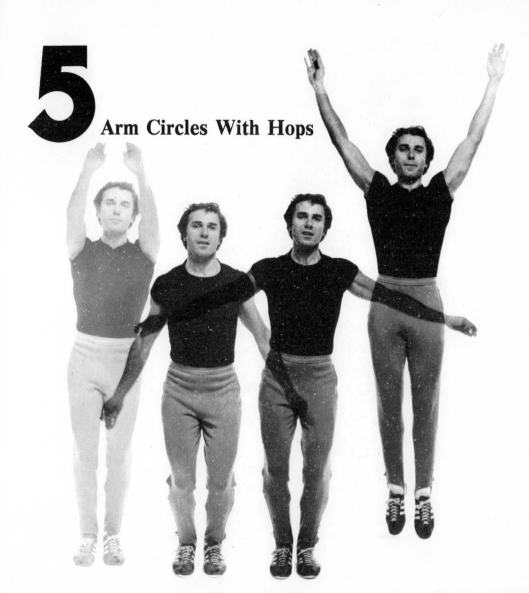

Draw wide circles with your arms on either side of the
body, keeping both arms "in step" with each other. This
exercise should be done very energetically. Accompany the
upward movement of the arms with a light hop. Repeat 10
to 15 times forward and 10 to 15 times in reverse.

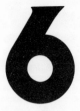 **Muscle Tension Exercise 1**

In a half squatting position, place left palm on the inside of the right knee, right palm on the inside of the left knee and press knees against palms. Hold the tension for 8 seconds (continue to breathe normally), then release. Repeat 3 times.

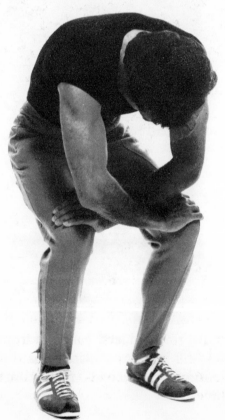

# 7 Muscle Tension Exercise 2

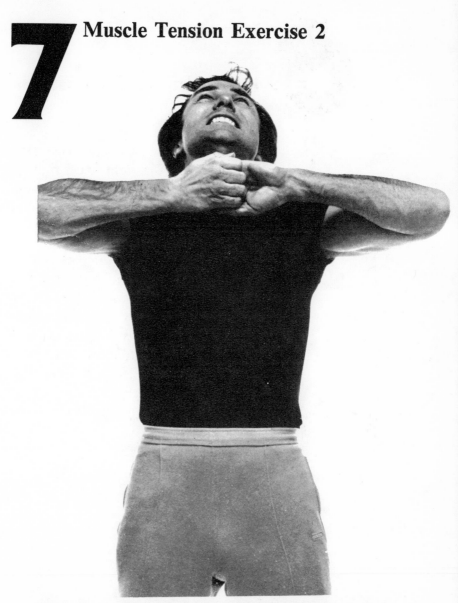

Elbows parallel to shoulders, hands in front of chest.
Clasp fingers and pull arms apart as hard as possible.
Hold the tension for 8 seconds, then relax the muscles.
Repeat 3 times.

# 8 Flexible Body Twists

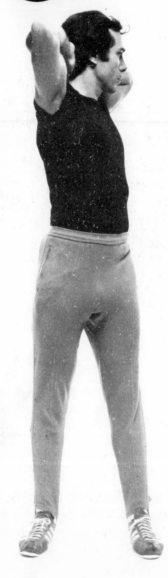

Stand firm, hands clasped behind head. Keeping legs fixed, vigorously twist the upper body from the hips ten times to the left and ten times to the right. Follow through, pulling elbows far back.

# 9 Twisting Body Bend

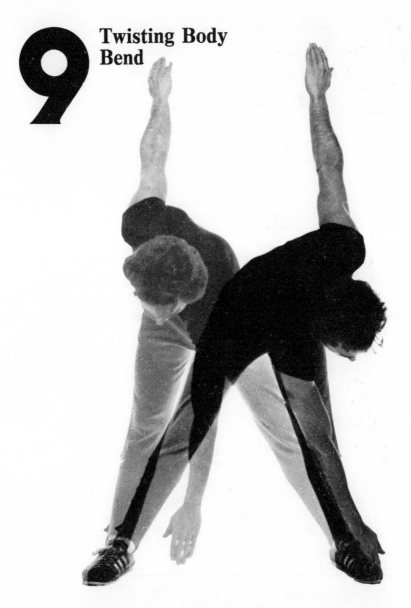

Legs apart, knees straight. Bending from the hips, touch left hand to right toe, right hand to left toe, ten times in each direction. Do this exercise rhythmically and breathe easily.

# 10 Alternating Body Bends

Legs apart, knees straight. Bending from the hips, touch fingers of both hands beyond the left foot, between the feet, and then beyond the right foot while exhaling. Then straighten up and inhale. Do this exercise rhythmically, ten times in a leftward direction and ten times in a rightward direction.

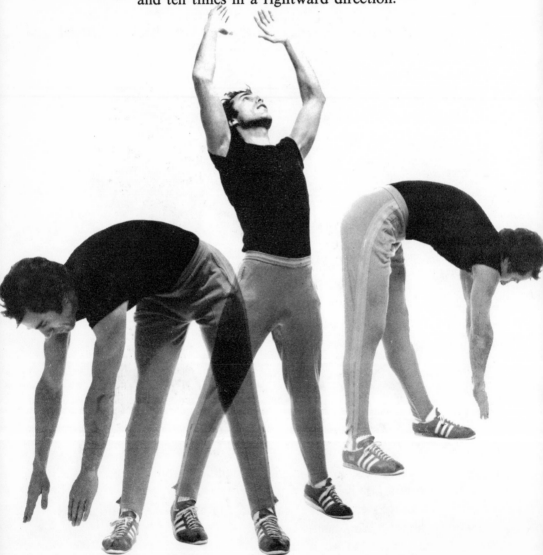

# 11 Jumping Jack

Starting from normal position, jump into a side straddle while raising arms sideways above the head and clapping hands. Immediately jump back to normal position. Repeat 10 to 20 times.

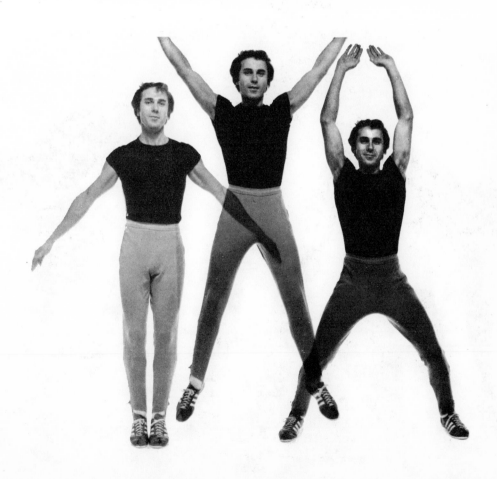

# 12 Hip Circles

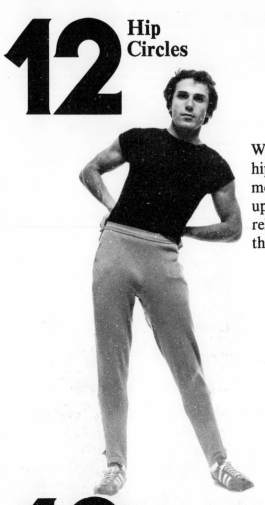

With legs apart and hands on hips, draw circular movements with the hips. The upper body should remain relaxed. Make ten circles to the left and ten to the right.

# 13 Knee Circles

With feet together and knees pressed together tightly, draw circular movements with your knees, ten times to the left and ten times to the right.

# 4. The Basic Calisthenic Exercises

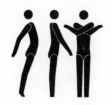

## 1 *Shoulder, Side, and Thigh Exercises*

*Starting position:* normal position, feet parallel.

*Tension:* Stretch body full length and lift arms sideways to form a 45° angle with the body. Draw arms backwards, stretching back, bottom, and leg muscles, and raising heels off the floor. At the height of tension turn the palms upwards.

*Release:* Relax back, bottom, and leg muscles and return heels to floor while simultaneously drawing outstretched arms forward from the shoulder, crossing them in front of the chest, and following through to the opposite side.

*Note:* Continue to breathe normally throughout the exercise; do not strain. Repeat 10 to 15 times.

(See basic exercise #1, page 38.)

49

# 2 *Stretching*

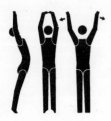

*Starting position:* normal position, feet parallel, arms
hanging loosely in front of body.

*Tension:* Clasp hands and while tensing all muscles raise
your hands directly in front of your body and over your
head. While doing this you should also be turning your
palms upward, raising your heels from floor and actively
extending the whole body to its maximum length. This
exercise is reminiscent of a stretching cat. Inhale deeply
while doing this.

*Release:* Relax the whole body, let arms fall to the sides in
wide arcs, and return to the starting position while
exhaling.

*Note:* Repeat this exercise 3 to 5 times.
(See basic exercise #2, page 39.)

# 3 *Tension—Release*

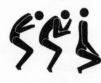

*Starting position:* legs slightly apart, feet parallel. Half
squatting position, knees should from an approximately
90° angle. Holding arms and fists in a boxing position in
front of chest, lean upper body forward, then raise and
arch the back backwards.

*Tension:* Tense all muscles and move the arms as if boxing
from the shoulders. Continue to breathe normally. Hold
the tension for about 6 to 8 seconds.

*Release:* Relax all muscles and fall into a deep squat. The
upper body should remain straight and the lower arms
rest relaxed on the thighs.

*Note:* Take 2 normal breaths before repeating this exercise,
and repeat for a total of 3 to 5 times.

# 4 *Sit and Stretch*

This exercise is a direct continuation of exercise 3 and leads over to exercise 5.

*Starting position:* A deep squat, upper body erect, back stretched, hands clasped behind head.

*Tension:* Inhale slowly while drawing elbows as far back as possible. The back muscles should be tightly stretched.

*Release:* While exhaling, relax the back muscles and bring the elbows slightly forward. Repeat the exercise 3 to 5 times.

*Note:* After that, unclasp your hands, and while bending the upper body forward, vigorously swing your arms down past your sides and behind your back. Simultaneously rise from the squatting position and return to the normal position.

# 5 *Breathing Exercise with Body Bend*

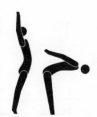

This exercise follows directly on exercise 4.

*Starting position:* legs slightly apart, feet parallel.

*Tension:* Inhale deeply while raising both arms above head and extending body to its maximum length.

*Release:* While exhaling, fall forward from hips, keeping upper body and knees stretched and straight. The arms will simultaneously fall forward. Follow through, drawing arms past and behind the sides of the body.

*Note:* The body should bend rather like a pocket knife at the hips. Straighten upper body while swinging arms back toward the front, returning to starting position. Repeat the exercise 10 to 15 times.

51

## 6 *Forward Shoulder Circles*

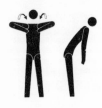

*Starting position:* same as #5. Hands under armpits, elbows parallel to shoulders. Roll the upper arm in forward circular movements from the shoulder joints.

*Tension:* The elbows will draw circles in the air. The top of the circle must lie above the shoulder level. Continue to breathe normally, do not strain. Repeat 10 to 15 times.

*Release:* Bend the upper body slightly forward from the starting position. This will relax the shoulder muscles. Shake out arms.

## 7 *Breathing Exercise with Sideward Body Bend*

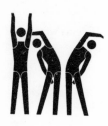

*Starting position:* legs slightly apart, feet parallel, arms above head.

*Tension:* Bend the body sidewards toward the left, breathe in, and let left arm swing behind body; return to starting position, bend body sidewards toward the right, breathe out, and let the right arm swing behind body.

*Note:* Repeat 5 times, then reverse, inhaling on the rightward bend and exhaling on the leftward bend. Repeat this version 5 times.

(See basic exercise #3, page 39.)

## 8 *Backward Shoulder Circles*

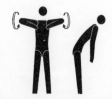

Same as exercise 6 except that the upper arms are rolled backwards (10 to 15 times), followed again by relaxing the shoulder muscles.

# 9  *Abdominal Breathing*

*Starting position:* legs slightly apart, feet parallel. Rest hands flatly on upper abdomen, that is, over the stomach. The upper body should be stretched.

*Tension:* While inhaling, push stomach outward against the slight resistance of the hands and while exhaling push hands against stomach. Repeat about 10 times.

# 10  *Forward Arm Circles with Hops*

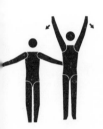

*Starting position:* normal position, feet parallel. Arms stretched to the side at shoulder height.

*Tension:* Draw wide backward circles with outstretched arms. The upward movement of the arms is accompanied by a gentle hopping from the ankles. Continue to breathe normally, do not strain.

*Note:* Repeat the exercise 10 times in the forward direction, then 10 times in the reverse direction. When finished, relax the shoulder muscles.

(See basic exercise #5, page 41.)

# 11  *Muscle Tensing Exercises*

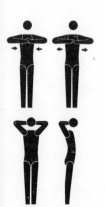

Of the nine tensing exercises that follow, three different ones should be performed three times a day every day.

In doing this exercise, it is important to hold the muscle tension at its highest level for about 8 seconds, relaxing the muscles afterwards. This is called isometric training.

*Note:* Continue to breathe normally even while tensing the muscles. It is very important that you do not hold your breath or strain your breathing.

a) Normal position, upright posture, elbows parallel to shoulders, hands in front of chest. Press the fist of one hand as hard as you can against the palm of the other.

b) Same position as in *a,* clasp fingers and pull arms apart as hard as possible (see basic exercise #7, page 43).

c) Normal position, upright posture, hands clasped behind head. Push hands forward against the resistance of the neck and back muscles, and hold for about 8 seconds.

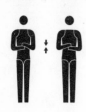

d) Normal position, upright posture, right palm on right temple, elbow at shoulder height. Press head and hand against each other as hard as possible.

e) Same as exercise *d,* this time with left hand and left temple

f) Normal position, upright posture. Bend arms at elbows, left wrist on top of right fist. Press one against the other as hard as possible in a vertical direction.

g) Same as exercise *f,* but this time with the right wrist on the left fist.

h) In a half squatting position, lean upper body forward, place left palm on the inside of the right knee, right palm on the inside of the left knee. Simultaneously press the knees against the palms (see basic exercise #6, page 42).

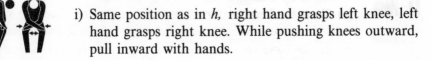

i) Same position as in *h,* right hand grasps left knee, left hand grasps right knee. While pushing knees outward, pull inward with hands.

# 12 *Deep Squat Body Bend*

*Starting position:* normal position, feet parallel, arms above the head. Breathe in deeply.
*Tension:* While exhaling, bend body forward and swing arms back and behind. Then return to the starting position via a deep squat and breathe in. Repeat 10 to 15 times.

# 13 *Arm Circles*

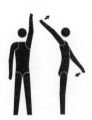

*Starting position:* legs slightly apart, feet parallel, left (or right) arm above head.
*Tension:* Circle both arms forward (similar to the crawl stroke in swimming), keeping arms straight and stretched, and pull through in strong strokes.
*Note:* Do the exercise 10 times in the forward direction and 10 times in the backward direction. Continue to breathe normally, do not strain.

# 14 *Neck Exercises*

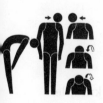

*Starting position:* normal position, arms straight, palms together between knees. Rotate shoulders as if rubbing palms together. This loosens neck and shoulder muscles. Stand up straight.
a) Turn the head as far as possible to the left, keeping your chin at the shoulder level. Looking leftward, bend neck forward and then backward as far as posssible. Do the exercises at a deliberately slow pace and do not jerk. Then do the same movements toward the right.
b) With the neck muscles as relaxed as possible, let the head fall forward, backward, to the left, and to the right.
c) Roll your head slowly several times toward the left and right, keeping your eyes open.

# 15 *Body Twists*

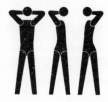

*Starting position:* legs apart, feet parallel, stand firm and
  straight, hands clasped behind head.
*Tension:* Keeping the pelvis in the normal position, twist the
  body toward the left and the right. Even better, twist the
  pelvis in the opposite direction to the body twist.
*Note:* Twist 10 times to the left and 10 times to the right.
  Continue to breathe normally, do not strain.
(See basic exercise #8, page 44.)

# 16 *Rocking Body Bends*

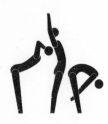

*Starting position:* same as exercise 15, hands clasped behind
  head.
*Tension:* Keeping upper body straight and tensing back
  muscles, let upper body fall forward from the hips and
  bounce. Return to starting position, raise arms above head
  and with relaxed back muscles let the upper body fall
  forward, the arms following smoothly as far as possible
  through the legs as if you wanted to reach an object that
  was lying some distance behind you. Return to starting
  position, hands clasped behind head.
*Note:* This exercise should be done energetically and
  rhythmically. Inhale each time you straighten up and
  exhale with the body bend. Do not hold your breath and
  do not strain. Repeat 5 to 10 times.

# 17 *Alternating Body Bends*

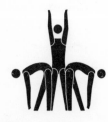

*Starting position:* legs apart, arms raised above head.
*Tension:* Bend trunk forward and to the left. The hands
  should touch the floor about 6 inches beyond the left foot,
  then between the feet and then 6 inches beyond the right
  foot. Stand up straight, lean backwards, and freeze. Bend

trunk forward and to the right and repeat the above
movement in the opposite direction.

*Note:* Breathe in while straightening up and exhale during
the body bend. Do the exercise rhythmically 10 times in
each direction. This exercise is relatively strenuous both
with regard to agility and condition. Touching the floor
on the far side of the feet might present difficulties for
you in the beginning. Do not force yourself, and do not
hold up your normal progress with this exercise. After a
while it will become automatic.

(See basic exercise #10, page 46.)

# 18 *Twisting Body Bend*

*Starting position:* legs apart, arms outstretched, body bent
forward from hips.

*Tension:* Keeping knees straight and arms outstretched,
twist body around touching left hand to right toe, and
vice versa. Do this exercise rhythmically, with 10 twists
to the left and 10 to the right.

*Note:* Continue to breathe normally, and above all, do not
strain. When finished, stand up and shake out arms and
legs.

(See basic exercise #9, page 45.)

# 19 *Hip Circles*

*Starting position:* legs apart, upper body erect, hands on
hips.

*Tension:* Keeping knees and back straight, circle the hips 10
times to the left and 10 times to the right.

*Note:* The circling movement should emanate only from the
hips.

(See basic exercise #12, page 48.)

# 20 *Knee Circles*

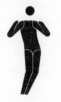

*Starting position:* tight normal position, feet together, toes
    pointed inward and lightly touching. Bend knees slightly.
*Tension:* Press knees together and make circular movements
    with them, 10 times to the left and 10 times to the right.
    This is a good warm-up exercise for skiers.
(See basic exercise #13, page 48.)

# 21 *Jumping Jack*

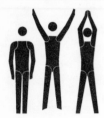

Starting from the normal position, jump into a side straddle
while raising arms sideways above the head and clapping
hands. Immediately jump back into the normal position.
Repeat 10 to 20 times.
(See basic exercise #11, page 47.)

# 22 *Loosening-up Exercise*

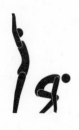

*Starting position:* normal position, arms above head,
    vigorously outstretched, all muscles strained, inhale. Now
    collapse, that is, sink into a deep squat and exhale.
    Maintain balance with the arms. Repeat 5 times.

    You can do these exercises wherever you find enough
room to move about, but if you have the opportunity, the
best place is outdoors in the fresh air (in the garden, on the
terrace, or balcony). If this is not possible, you should
exercise near an open window.
    If you live in an apartment house, the jumping exercises
may disturb your neighbors. You can alleviate this problem
by using a mat or a folded blanket.

*Study the individual steps of the exercises carefully and make sure you perform them exactly. You can control this more easily if you practice in front of a large mirror. Only after you have mastered the individual exercises should you attempt to do the whole program in sequence.*

After a few weeks the proper performance of the exercises will be so securely anchored in your mind that you will no longer need to consult this book.

Now to the question as to what success can be expected from this kind of calisthenics program if you do the exercises regularly. As their name indicates, the "basic calisthenics" are designed to establish a firm base. A healthy support system—as defined above—is a prerequisite for any athletic activity. Not only does it bear the brunt of every training program, it is also what makes a continuous stress possible in the first place.

*Better agility through gymnastics*

*The basic calisthenic exercises are primarily directed toward strengthening the muscles, tendons and ligaments, and improving the mobility of the joints.*

Moreover, this results in a whole series of positive and very welcome side effects having to do with metabolism, respiration, and the circulatory functions in addition to the psychological benefits. To what extent your heart will be taxed by these exercises and its functioning improved depends upon several factors:
- its current productive capacity
- the intensity, and that means primarily the pace, at which you do the exercises, and
- the pulse rate you reach during the exercise
- the length of time you maintain the effective stress in training.

Yet, an essential, or for our purposes sufficient, improvement of your endurance capacity cannot be attained in this way. This is not to say, however, that the exercises have absolutely no effect in heightening your endurance. Your endurance can be improved through the so-called conditioning calisthenics which, by easily combining the individual parts of the exercises and increasing the exercise pace, turn the gymnastic elements into suitable exercises for an improvement of one's endurance.

# Conditioning Calisthenics

*Conditioning calisthenics use the gymnastic elements of the exercises to improve a person's endurance capacity by combining the individual parts of the exercises with an increased pace.*

Exercises that require special equipment (gymnastic ball, medicine ball, bars, ropes, etc.) as well as those that do not, are suitable. The variety of exercises that these objects produce is at once the advantage and the disadvantage of the method. On the one hand, the whole body and the heart are exercised at the same time. The exercises never become boring. On the other hand, this type of program requires so much previous knowledge and skills that in order to do it correctly one must either be a physical educator himself or be supervised by one. For this reason the conditioning calisthenics are primarily suited for group exercises under the direction of an experienced instructor. Yet, individual parts of the exercises can also be successfully integrated into your own exercise program.

*Especially suited for group exercises*

Jump ropes, for example, are particularly popular as a training apparatus, especially among boxers. Yet, even exercises without special equipment can be combined to produce particularly effective results. For the inexperienced, the difficulty lies, aside from mastering the repertoire, in properly controlling the pace and the intensity of the exercise.

# Aerobic Endurance and Pulse Rate

*Crucial for an improvement of one's general aerobic endurance is*
- *the stress that dynamic work places on the circulatory system*
- *with an intensity that leads to a certain pulse rate and*
- *which is sustained for at least 6 minutes.*

The type of stress is unimportant here, provided it is of a dynamic nature. The number of heart beats per minute—the pulse rate—thus gains a particular importance in determining the intensity of the stress.

We all know that our heart beats more quickly when we exert ourselves physically. Yet, it not only beats more quickly, but more strongly as well—this is called heart palpitations. This is completely normal and is a sign that our heart has to perform more work because the working muscle needs more oxygen and therefore "uses up" more blood. (see the chapter on "Basic Knowledge," p. 111, for more details about this.) Other things being equal, and if the accelerated heart activity is produced by the work itself, the number of heart beats per minute is a measure of the intensity of the stress. (There are also others, for example, emotional reasons for "palpitations", but we will not go into them here.)

*Measurement of stress intensity*

*We can use the number of heart beats per minute, in other words the pulse rate, to determine whether a dynamic physical stress is intensive enough to produce a training effect on the heart.*

You will recall that the number 170 minus your age gives the pulse rate at which you can expect a positive training effect. Specialists in the field call this number the minimum training pulse rate.

61

In the case of a 44-year-old person, a dynamic activity has to produce a pulse rate of *at least* 126/min. if it is to be effective. Since this is a minimum or lower limit, I recommend for healthy individuals a pulse rate of at least 180 minus their age, that is, the number resulting from 180 minus your age rounded off to the next higher ten.

*Ascertaining your training rate*

I call this number the *adjustment rate* because it enables you to adjust the intensity of the stress accordingly. For example: you are 44 years old and would like to ascertain your training rate. 180 minus 44 gives 136, rounded off to the next higher ten, 140. To be effective for you, an activity must therefore produce a pulse rate of about 140 beats per minute. You are "within range" if your pulse beats between 130 and 150 times per minute during the performance phase (I will return to this point later).

The question is, how can you determine this? The easiest way is by counting; if you want to have it even easier, you can use a small instrument.

To take your pulse, you need a clock, preferably one with a second hand. The best place to count your pulse during stress is on the left or right side of the neck. Practice this a bit so that you can find the correct place automatically.

*The 15-second-count*

*Count the number of pulse beats for 15 seconds and multiply this amount by 4. The result is your pulse rate, accurate to within 4 beats.*

This degree of accuracy is adequate. For our purposes, all you really need to know is your 15-second-count; the multiplication is unnecessary. That means, to continue our previous example, that the pulse of a 44-year-old person has to beat about 35 times, but no less than 32 times, within 15 seconds if the exercise is to be effective.

There are small battery operated instruments you can buy that will electronically determine your heart or pulse rate based on what are called heart action potentials*. These

---

* bioelectrical phenomena during muscle contraction

instruments indicate on a small scale or with an optical or acoustical signal whether the heart rate is within a previously chosen range.

The heart action potentials are then conducted to the instrument. This is accomplished by two electrodes fastened to a belt worn around the chest and linked to the instrument by thin wires. These instruments are comfortable and, when used correctly, relatively safe to operate and reliable, but unfortunately they are very expensive.

The chart on page 64 lists and explains the activities with a view toward their proper, that is, their training effective execution. When performed systematically and appropriately, these activities are almost equivalent in their effect. They all lead to a sustained exertion beyond the endurance limit and thus represent a functional stimulant for the improvement of one's endurance capacity.

Choose one of the following endurance activities that corresponds to your inclinations and available facilities. Naturally you can also combine two or more of them. But, since there is nothing that would represent only advantages (or only disadvantages), each of these activities also involves certain prerequisites or conditions that you will have to take into account before making your decision.

This chart shows that there is unfortunately no "ideal" endurance sport. Each of these activities has aggravating even if different "double edges," so that you are probably not yet able to decide which represents the lesser evil in your individual case. You may find the choice easier after you read the next chapter.

*Is your favorite sport included?* Many of you will probably miss your favorite sport, such as tennis, golf, or riding, in this list of activities. This does not mean that I would like to discourage you from participating in these activities in the future. On the contrary, every sport that provides enjoyment and an opportunity to offset the strain of your daily life in a natural way will contribute to an improvement of your well-being and therefore has its own positive effect.

Precise scientific tests, however, have clearly indicated

# Choose Your Own Training Activity

(Consult the "Decision Table" on p. 105 to find out which activity is best suited to you.)

| Activity | Prerequisite | Time Investment | Skills | Greatest Advantage | Greatest Disadvantage |
|---|---|---|---|---|---|
| **Cycling** | healthy back | slight | everyone can learn, no special skills | almost no prerequisites | dependent upon the weather, traffic danger |
| **Exercise Bicycle** | ergometer is expensive | slight | not necessary | stress can be precisely measured | boring |
| **Conditioning Calisthenics** | no serious physical handicaps | slight | almost always need supervision by a trained coach | manysided, the whole body is trained | difficult to do without a coach |
| **Hiking** | appropriate landscape, hills, healthy legs | great, at least one hour a day required | not necessary | communing with nature | requires a considerable amount of time |
| **Running** | weight normal legs and back healthy | slight | none | independence, is fun, no danger from traffic | not suited for everyone |
| **Swimming** | swimming pool with free lane | relatively great | very strenuous, you must be able to swim correctly | no static stress | most people lack the proper skills |
| **Rowing** | water, boat, crew | great | slight | increases strength and endurance | most people lack the prerequisites |
| **Rowing Machines** | rowing machine | slight | none | same as for rowing | boring |

that only the activities described in this book have a demonstrable influence on general aerobic endurance. Since a good overall endurance is an essential prerequisite for good performance in any sport, top athletes in all fields regularly practice a compensatory or conditioning training to improve their endurance capacity. The greatest popularity here seems to go particularly to long distance activities and conditioning calisthenics, including the jump rope.

You will soon notice that your favorite sport will provide much more pleasure once you have improved your stamina.

# 5. Cycling

*Racing cyclists, especially cross-country cyclists, are among those athletes with the greatest overall aerobic endurance. That is why cycling is particularly suited even for non-professionals for improving their endurance capacity.*

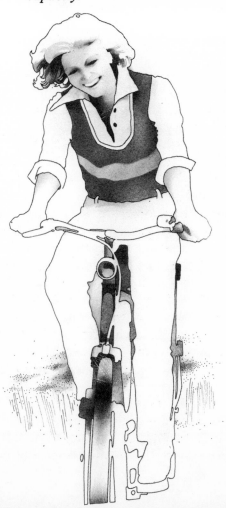

*The advantages of cycling*

The advantages of this sport are numerous and diverse:
- the individual cyclist can determine the limit of the stress on the circulation and thus just about dictate the results of his endurance training.
- It is almost impossible, particularly for the inexperienced, to genuinely overexert themselves, because only a relatively small group of muscles is involved and these "tire" sooner than the heart does.
- Very few physical skills are required; almost anyone can ride a bicycle.
- The mechanical stress on the suppport system is minimal, the body weight is supported by the saddle and even mobility handicaps (such as limited mobility resulting from accidents, injuries, or illnesses) represent no absolute hindrance.
- Cycling is the only sport that can be combined easily and inconspicuously with practical needs. The training can be done—at least in many cases—on the way to work.
- Biking can be pursued just as well alone as in the company of family or friends.
- The technical prerequisites are modest: everyone can afford a bicycle, even a good one.
- You can ride almost anywhere.

I know of only two drawbacks: bicycling is dependent upon the weather and presents a danger of accident in heavy traffic. Yet, these should not be overestimated. Certainly whoever lives in a large metropolitan area cannot avoid the traffic, and 8 inches of snow do represent a considerable handicap. On the other hand, however, the old adage is also true: there is no bad weather, only inappropriate clothing; and, where there is a will, there is a way—this time quite literally meant. Usually "weather" and "traffic" are only a welcome excuse to occasionally leave the bicycle at home out of pure laziness.

*Tips for aspiring cyclists*

Here are a few tips for aspiring cyclists: if you want to buy a bicycle as a training tool, choose a model with the lightest possible frame and the largest possible wheels. Folding bicycles are practical to take along, but impractical to ride.

Changeable gears are also to be recommended. They enable you to ride constantly at an optimal number of pedal revolutions, which should be relatively high (60-80 pedal rpm).

Make a note of the following basic rule: the higher the number of pedal revolutions per minute, the greater the stress.

*Adjust saddle height properly*

*The most frequent mistake "occasional" riders make is to adjust the saddle incorrectly, usually too low. The height of the saddle is correctly fixed when the working leg is fully stretched to reach the pedal at its lowest point. In so doing, the knee is not completely straight, but should form an angle of about 160°.*

The second most frequent mistake: either the toes or the arch of the foot rests upon the pedal (an indirect consequence of an incorrect saddle height). The ball of the foot of the working leg should rest on the pedal with relaxed muscles when the pedal is at its lowest point. Only in this way will you be able to fully employ the calf muscles.

With many people one leg is shorter than the other. In this case it pays to shorten the appropriate pedal shank.

Mass produced bicycles almost always vary in the size of their frames. You should choose a make whose frame size best corresponds to your body build. An equalization can be attained by adjusting the handlebars.

The following basic rules also apply for cycling: take your time in the beginning and keep warm. The part of the body that receives the second greatest strain is the buttocks. A 10-minute ride daily is better than to attempt a *tour de force* on weekends.

*Training schedule*

*The way to proceed is:*
● *dress appropriately for training*

69

- *fix or check the height of the saddle*
- *take and record your pulse*
- *ride slowly at first*
- *gradually increase the stress so that you reach your training pulse rate after about 5 minutes (warm up)*
- *ride at "full" speed for another minute or so*
- *then gradually reduce the stress in such a way that your pulse rate always remains near the adjustment rate (see above) plus or minus 10 beats\* (performance phase)*
- *If you train daily, ride for a total of about 10 minutes within range of the performance phase. If you train only 4 times a week, you should extend the performance phase to about 20 minutes each time.*
- *Gradually reduce the stress so that after about 5 minutes you are riding at a strolling pace. Your pulse rate should have fallen by at least 20 beats a minute (wind down).*
- *Divide your training route in such a way that you are back home again by the end of the wind down phase.*

*Beware of catching cold*

If you have done it correctly, you will be perspiring heavily. It is therefore important not to stretch out the wind down phase much beyond five minutes, for you could catch a cold, even in the summer. If you find you have miscalculated the time or the distance, and have not reached home after five minutes of wind down, it is better to increase your speed again than to continue "strolling" along.

Prolonging the performance phase beyond the given time periods is not only harmless, it also increases the effect. At the beginning of your training, though, you should try to adhere to the time schedule as closely as possible. You yourself will notice why: a muscle cramp cannot be completely avoided.

---

\* The pulse rate has a "dragging effect," which means that it adjusts to the stress with a temporary delay (one to five minutes). This is why it remains high even when the intensity of the stress is reduced.

70

To summarize: in the beginning of your training
- train daily
- 5 minute warm up, 10 minute performance, 5 minute wind down
- take a long hot shower immediately after training, and avoid cold water under all circumstances. Put on a complete change of clothes, or at least a fresh pair of dry underwear.

*Ride out muscle cramps*

If you get a muscle cramp—and you surely will get one if you have not previously ridden a bicycle on a regular basis—that should be no reason for you to discontinue your training. You have to ride the cramp out, for this is the quickest way to relieve it. And always obey the rule of straining only so hard during the performance phase that your pulse rate lies within 10 beats of the adjustment rate.

While doing this, you will probably notice that your performance capacity apparently decreases during the first two weeks of training. You reach your training effective rate with a perceptibly lower stress level than on the first or second day of training. This is normal and need not disturb you. Specialists call this the muscular adaptation phenomenon. However, if your pulse rate at rest is clearly higher (you should record it before every training session), if it becomes irregular or if any heart trouble develops, you should consult your physician.

# Ergometer Training

A special form of cycling is training on "home trainers", which is another name for exercise bicycles or ergometers\*. I recommend this apparatus only in exceptional cases.

*Stationary bicycles*

Why? Because there is probably nothing more absurd than riding a bicycle and never getting anywhere. This is why many exercise bicycles end up in the basement after a few weeks and produce, not well-being, but only a bad conscience instead. Yet, this only applies to "weak-willed" —or, better, not sufficiently motivated—individuals, and surely you are not one of these.

When looked at objectively, ergometers have the same advantages that normal bicycles do without the disadvantages. The rider is not affected by the weather and is not endangered by street traffic. If you would like to use such a machine, then please make sure that it has as large a flywheel as possible. Most of the models on the market today do not meet this requirement. It is important for the following reason: I have already explained that a stress that is effective in training and which is supposed to improve one's overall endurance has to be dynamic, and therefore has to be combined with movement. In addition, it also has to be sufficiently intensive. Only when both are together and combined with a sufficiently long period of stress can a training effect be guaranteed.

On a normal bicycle the intensity of the stress can be

---

\* *Ergometer:* work or performance gauge. An instrument for the quantitative measurement of physical stress, such as a treadmill ergometer or a bicycle ergometer (a special type of exercise bicycle). Unlike most exercise bikes, a good ergometer measures braking resistance as well as the speed of the pedal revolutions per minute in precise numerical quantities. Only an ergometer can measure performance, thus it makes a measurable, controllable and reproducible training possible for healthy people, and, when used under a physician's direction, is also suitable for heart patients. Moreover, only an ergometer permits what is called the conditioning test, and this can be an incentive for daily training.

varied at will very simply by choosing the gear and speed. With an exercise bicycle this can only be done with the help of a brake. If there is no flywheel, the dynamics are impaired; the wheel stops when you stop pedalling. In this way the stress acquires a predominantly static character (similar to that in stretching chest expanders or in lifting weights), and the desired effect is lost, indeed it can even result in harmful side effects.

*Flywheel produces dynamics*

Before you buy one of these bicycles, check whether the flywheel is large enough. You can determine this without the aid of any tools and without having to rely on the assurances of the salesperson or recommendations from friends: simply set the brake at a medium level of stress and ride it at 80 pedal rpm for a short time; ten pedal revolutions will do. If you now stop pedalling, the wheel has to continue to rotate for a short time. In any case, it should not stop the very moment you stop pedalling.

*What to check before buying an exercise bicycle*

Another point you should take into consideration is that the stress should be measurable. Two things have to be kept in mind here:
● the number of pedal revolutions per minute or the fictitious riding speed;
● the strength of the braking action.

Most exercise bicycles are only equipped with an indicator, usually a gauge called a tachometer, to measure the number of revolutions. The scale to which the bicycles are calibrated is completely irrelevant. The only thing that is essential is that both functions are given (braking resistance and pedal revolutions). The amount of stress, the performance, in other words, that you produce with the machine is computed as the product of the pedal speed and the braking resistance.

Just to be complete, I should mention that there are machines that indicate the performance directly (usually in watts), or machines that let you choose and set the desired performance beforehand. With a bicycle of this kind, one can make do with only one indicator.

These ergometers are used especially in medical

examinations. They cost as much as a medium priced automobile and are thus out of the question for private use as a training apparatus.

The stress should also be reproducible. Therefore, you not only have to be able to reliably read the pedal speed and the braking resistance, but also be able to set it exactly. This is the only way to fully realize the decisive advantage this training apparatus has over others—namely, the ability to set the precise stress dosage.

Another thing you should require is that the saddle and handle bars be easily and freely adjustable, without pre-set positions. The saddle especially has to be able to be raised far enough so as to attain a favorable efficiency level of the working muscles.

What I have already said about the height of the saddle and the position of the foot for riding a bicycle outdoors obviously also applies to riding an exercise bicycle.

If you have decided to use an exercise bicycle to improve your condition, then the following pages will be of particular interest to you because they will tell you how to do this type of training. Simply riding a bicycle is not enough. You have to do it correctly.

Although I have already explained the basic principle above, I want to repeat it once again: to be effective, an exercise has to be maintained at an appropriate degree of intensity for a certain minimum amount of time.

As far as the length of an effective stress is concerned, I have already indicated that six minutes represent a minimum and that the effect can be clearly increased by increasing the duration of the exercise.

*This is why I recommend a performance phase of 10 minutes for daily training, 20 minutes each session when you train only 4 times a week, and as a "maintenance dose" 30 minutes twice a week.*

The ergometer training program

Follow this procedure in your training program:
- wear an appropriate training outfit
- set or check the saddle height
- measure your pulse rate and record it
- start riding at first without any braking resistance and increase the speed to 55 pedal rpm
- set the braking resistance at .5 kp (braking resistance is most frequently measured in kiloponds = kp)
- pedal for 1 minute at this stress

*Warm up*

- increase the speed to 60 pedal rpm and pedal for 1 minute (30 watts)
- increase the braking resistance to 1.0 kp and pedal for 1 minute (60 watts)
- during the last 15 seconds of this minute, take your pulse rate and compare it to your 15-second-count.
- If you have not yet reached your training pulse rate, increase the speed to 65 pedal rpm and pedal for 1 minute.
- increase the braking resistance by .5 kp to 1.5 kp and pedal for 1 minute
- during the last 15 seconds of this minute, take your pulse and compare it with your 15-second-count.

Now increase speed by 5 pedal rpm, pedal for 1 minute, increasing braking resistance by .5 kp, pedal for 1 minute, and during the last 15 seconds take your pulse and continue in this way until you have reached your adjustment rate (180 minus your age), rounded off to the next highest 10. You have now warmed up and have reached the performance phase, which in a daily training program should last 10 minutes.

*10 minute performance phase*

Performance phase:
- increase the braking resistance again by .5 kp and ride for 1 minute

- now reduce the braking resistance by 1 kp and ride for 1 minute
- during the last 15 seconds, measure your pulse rate and compare it with your 15-second-count. By now it must be within 10 pulse beats of your adjustment rate.
- If this is the case, increase the braking resistance again by 1 kp, ride for 1 minute, then reduce by 1 kp, ride for another minute, and count your pulse during the last 15 seconds.
- Alternate in this way for 10 minutes, keeping the number of pedal rpm in the same range of braking resistance at which you reached your training rate.

You can picture the effect of this kind of interval stress (which, by the way, is not to be confused with interval training), in the following way: you will recall that we have defined training as measured doses of overexertion. In this, the working muscles are not sufficiently supplied with enough energy carriers and oxygen. The energy producing processes of muscle metabolism are therefore increasingly converted from the purely aerobic (dependent upon oxygen) to the anaerobic (not dependent upon oxygen) "production method." Metabolic wastes are produced which can be called "fatigue elements."

When these fatigue elements reach a certain level of concentration, the energy producing process is automatically reduced, that is, the energy producing process slows down in direct proportion to the increasing concentration of fatigue elements. The muscles have incurred an oxygen debt; in other words, because of the oxygen supply, they have used up more energy than was actually at their disposal. They "have lived beyond their means" (overexertion).

As every debt in everyday life always carries a burden of interest, the organism too has to pay off the "oxygen interest" in addition to its oxygen debt. This can be done only through a corresponding heart activity. This is why the heart activity and with it the pulse rate remain high for a while even after the stress has been reduced. Therefore, you should administer your "highs" and "rests" in proper doses

76

so that your heart rate always remains within the training effective range (the calculated training rate plus or minus 10).

● Should your pulse rate rise again and exceed the value of the adjustment rate plus 10 at the end of the "recovery stage", then you can reduce the level by .5 kp; however, you should maintain the speed.

Example: You are 44 years old. Your adjustment rate is accordingly 140/min., the training effective pulse rate range therefore lies between 130 and 150 beats per minute. You have reached your training rate at 1.5 kp and 65 pedal rpm and you will pedal in one minute intervals between 1.0 kp (recovery stage) and 2.0 kp (performance stage) at 65 pedal rpm. Let's assume that at the end of the 6th minute of the performance phase your measured 15-second-count amounted to 40, which is 160 pulse beats per minute. At this time you can reduce the level by .5 kp, and then alternate between .5 and 1.5 kp.

Your pulse rate will then calm down a bit. You will probably have trouble with your legs sooner than with your pulse rate and you will soon realize the reason for alternating the stress. If your legs can bear it, it is by no means dangerous if your pulse rate goes beyond the upper limit (adjustment rate plus or minus 10) as long as you do not reach the value of 220 minus your age. Even then there is no danger: but neither do you gain any further advantage.

*Wind down* ● At the end of the performance phase (after 10 minutes of interval stress), reduce the stress the same way you increased it during the warm up, simply in the opposite direction:

● reduce the braking resistance by .5 kp, ride for 1 minute, reduce the speed by 5 pedal rpm, ride for 1 minute

● and so on until you have arrived at 0 kp braking resistance (wind down).

This winding down is very important and by no means a waste of time. With it you attain a better circulation to the muscles, and a quicker removal of the fatigue elements. It also minimizes the possibility of a Charley horse.

● Observe the safety tips on page 32 during and after the stress.

● Check your pulse rate again one hour after you have ended your training session. If your pulse has not calmed down by then, you should consult your physician.

*Here is a summary of the important points:*
● *check the height of the saddle*
● *determine your pulse rate*
● *start riding without any braking resistance*
● *set the speed at 55 pedal rpm*
● *when stress reaches .5 kp, the warm up period begins.*
● *In one minute intervals increase the speed by 5 pedal rpm and the braking resistance by .5 kp and take your pulse rate during the last 15 seconds.*
● *Continue to increase until you reach the adjustment rate.*
● *Increase the resistance by .5 kp (beginning of the performance phase) and ride for 1 minute.*
● *Reduce the resistance by 1.0 kp and ride for 1 minute—take your pulse during the last 15 seconds.*
● *During the performance phase, alternate the braking resistance in this way in 1 minute intervals.*
● *If your pulse is climbing, reduce the stress level by .5 kp but keep the speed constant.*
● *To wind down, reduce alternatingly the braking resistance by .5 kp and the speed by 5 pedal rpm in one minute intervals until you reach 0 braking resistance.*

If you do your training in this way and choose the stress during the performance phase in such a way that your pulse rate always remains within the previously calculated training effective range, the training load will conform autodynamically to your current degree of fitness, will equalize the fluctuations in your daily performance and will bring about a gradual improvement of your endurance capacity.

# 6. Running

*Running is one of the nicest and most effective ways to increase your endurance capacity. Moreover, it is the sport with the least technical and geographical prerequisites. It does not demand a great deal of time, costs nothing, and is affected by neither traffic nor bad weather.*

For me, running represents stamina in its purest form. It is the most natural form of movement. It can do the same for you if you heed these three prerequisites:

*Is your support system in order?*

- your weight must be normal, or, if not, you have to bring it to its normal level before beginning your training.
- you have to have healthy feet, legs, knees and ankles, and
- your back cannot be giving you any trouble. Running is the stamina building discipline that makes the highest mechanical claim upon your support system because with every step each leg is called upon to brake a kinetic energy equal to the gravitational pull of your body weight falling from a height of about 8 inches.

Defective or injured joints, weak ligaments, or arch defects usually lead to problems while running which very quickly render the training impossible. Problems with your spine and discs are other constitutional conditions that prove to be incompatible with jogging over the long run.

Yet, even if your support system is in order, it will not remain that way for long if you are overweight when you begin your training. The forces that running exerts upon your bones, joints, muscles, ligaments, and tendons will very shortly render even the healthiest feet unusable.

As long as you do not meet these requirements, or if they cannot be satisfied because of constitutional reasons, you should choose a different sport, such as cycling or swimming, for instance. If, however, your weight is normal and your bones healthy, I consider long distance running the ideal training method for you. This is as true for men as for women. I find the neglect of long distance running in women's sports incomprehensible, since women in general possess better constitutional requirements for running than men do. They have comparatively longer legs and less weight.

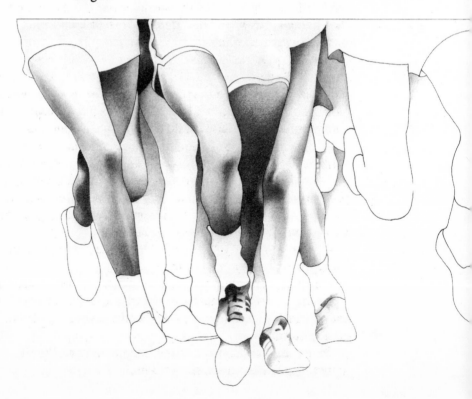

82

Age *per se* does not represent any hindrance either in attaining good or even internationally recognized skills in endurance races. I am not saying this to arouse your olympic ambitions, but rather to dispel an unfounded and yet widespread misconception.

*Two rules are of particular importance especially for older aspirants:*
- *start out slowly and*
- *keep warm.*

What does "start out slowly" mean in running? You can ride a bicycle, row, swim or do gymnastic exercises slowly without getting out of breath, but running is running and—even at the slowest pace—the inexperienced very soon finds himself "out of breath". Everyone knows this from personal experience. Remember: all good things in their time. A good way to start, then, is to talk about the necessary preparations.

Review what we have said on page 26 about proper training clothing. In running, naturally, having the correct shoes is of primary importance. Always wear socks when you run. If your feet blister easily, you should powder them and wear thin cotton socks under heavy woolen ones.

In the beginning you should take particular care in looking for a suitable path. It should be flat and even, but not paved, and free of all obstacles. Well-kept forest or park pathways are ideal. Later, when you have gotten used to running, this is no longer so important, and then you can run wherever there is enough room.

*Running as a training program*
We are now ready to set up a schedule. This program is based on the following principles:
- We shall gradually increase the effective performance until we reach a level of long-term endurance in keeping with our own current productive capacity while paying particular attention to
- the gradual adaptation of the support organs (bones, joints, ligaments, muscles, and tendons).

This is approximately the way one would formulate it in scientific terms. In plain English it means that you should lengthen your running distance only to the extent to which your heart and your support organs allow and only to the point that you can maintain a running pace over hills and dales for 20 to 30 minutes and still perceive it as "relaxation". This will not happen overnight, and it takes longer for some than for others. Even so, it is within reach of everyone.

- whose heart is healthy (consult a physician)
- whose weight is normal and
- who has healthy bones.

The program is divided into three phases:

## Outline of running program

*First phase*    **Preprogram:** goal-oriented exercises—running (see p. 86).

*Second*         **Build up Program:**
*phase*             *Method:* interval run
                *Duration of training session:* increasing up to 30 minutes
                *Frequency:* 6 times a week, later 4 times a week
                *Goal:* an endurance run of up to 30 minutes with active pauses

| Step | Part I: Warmup | Part II: Training Program | Part III: Rest |
|---|---|---|---|
| 1 | goal-oriented exercises | alternate 20DS running with 80DS walking in 10 minute intervals | goal-oriented exercises |
| 2 | goal-oriented exercises | alternate 30DS running with 70DS walking in 10 minute intervals | goal-oriented exercises |
| 3 | goal-oriented exercises | alternate 40DS running with 60DS walking in 10 minute intervals | goal-oriented exercises |
| 4 | goal-oriented exercises | alternate 50DS running with 50DS walking in 10 minute intervals | goal-oriented exercises |
| 5 | goal-oriented exercises | alternate 60DS running with 40DS walking in 10 minute intervals | goal-oriented exercises |
| 6 | goal-oriented exercises | alternate 70DS running with 30DS walking in 10 minute intervals | goal-oriented exercises |
| 7 | goal-oriented exercises | alternate 80DS running with 20DS walking in 10 minute intervals | goal-oriented exercises |
| 8 | goal-oriented exercises | alternate 90DS running with 10DS walking in 10 minute intervals | goal-oriented exercises |
| 9 | goal-oriented exercises | run for 10 minutes | goal-oriented exercises |
| 10 | goal-oriented exercises | run for 12 minutes | goal-oriented exercises |
| 11 | goal-oriented exercises | run for 14 minutes | goal-oriented exercises |
| 12 | goal-oriented exercises | run for 16 minutes | goal-oriented exercises |

From now on you only need train 4 times a week.

| Step | Part I: Warmup | Part II: Training Program | Part III: Rest |
|---|---|---|---|
| 13 | goal-oriented exercises | run for 18 minutes | goal-oriented exercises |
| 14 | goal-oriented exercises | run for 20 minutes | goal-oriented exercises |
| 15 | goal-oriented exercises | run for 30 minutes with 2 to 3 walking pauses | goal-oriented exercises |

*DS = double step; each time the left foot hits the ground counts as one step (1DS)

**Maintenance Program:**
   *Method:* long distance run with active rests (walking pauses)
   *Duration:* about 30 minutes
   *Frequency:* twice a week
   *Goal:* maintaining the endurance capacity

Follow step 15 of the Build up Program twice a week.

## Phase I: Pre-program

In running, the joint that is trained the most is the ankle, which connects the foot to the lower part of the leg, or better said, the joint that separates the leg from the foot. The muscles that are subjected to the greatest strain are those of the lower leg and primarily the calf muscle with its achilles tendon.

*Goal-oriented exercises for running*

*For those who are starting to run for the first time, especially older people, and also for those who have not run for a long time, it is very important that you do not suddenly burden your joints and muscles with a great stress, but rather prepare them gradually and systematically.*

This is why you should supplement your basic program with the following exercises.

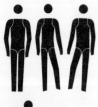

### 1. Strengthening the Calf Muscles
Normal starting position, feet parallel, toes pointed slightly inward. Rise up alternatingly on the left and then the right toes while shifting your whole body weight to the corresponding left or right leg. Sink down slowly and repeat 10 to 20 times.

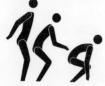

### 2. Stretching Exercise
Go from the normal position into a deep squat. While

86

keeping heels as flat as possible on the ground, shift your weight slightly forward and bounce or seesaw a few times. Repeat 3 to 5 times.

### 3. Shake Out Your Legs

### 4. Strengthening the Ankles
Hop lightly with both feet from the ankles, keeping the knees relaxed and slightly bent. This exercise could be described as jumping rope without the rope, although you could use one if you so desired. Repeat 10 to 50 times.

### 5. Stretching Exercise
Normal position, feet parallel and close together, knees straight. Bend body forward and grasp the calf in the region of the achilles tendon. Pull the upper body vigorously toward the legs while keeping knees straight. Repeat 5 to 10 times.

### 6. Shake Out Your Legs

### 7. Easy Running On The Spot
Do 50 to 100 DS. The feet must be raised 6 to 8 inches from the ground. Land on the balls of your feet and follow through until the heels touch the ground. In so doing, you must maintain the same foot position described in exercise 1.

### 8. Shake Out Your Legs
When you can do all of these preparatory exercises in the recommended dosage without straining and without getting out of breath, you are ready for

## Phase II: Build up program

*Desired goal, getting used to running*

*The primary goal of the build up program is to adapt the support system to the muscles, tendons, ligaments,*

87

*joints and bones that are subjected to particular strain during running. This serves to reduce the strain on your heart.*

In every training program, the support system is the "middle man". This is why it is also your most important tool. If this tool is not in order, you cannot continue to train. Therefore you should do the steps exactly as described in Phase II, and only go on after the transition criteria have been completely satisfied, even if you are convinced that you can already (or still) do much more.

The transition criteria are:
● your pulse rate at the end of the so-called performance phase of each training session,
● the current condition of your "running tools".

The build up program is subdivided into 15 steps which differ from one another in the length of the walking intervals and running time.

Each of these steps has three parts:
1) The first part serves to get you used to the movement while at the same time warming you up.
2) The second part is the actual training effective phase. We can therefore call it the performance phase.
3) In the third part, the stress is reduced and your heart and muscles should begin to calm down.

The transition from one constructive stage to the next higher one is triggered by the transition criteria mentioned above. Only after they have been met can you attempt the next step.

● At the end of the performance phase, your pulse rate must be within your own training effective range.
● You cannot run if you have any trouble with your feet or your legs (and absolutely not if you have any heart trouble).

*Warm up* **Build Up Program, Step 1, Part 1**
Modify the goal-oriented exercises for running, since you will be doing these to a certain extent during the walking pauses.

88

● Walk at a brisk pace for 100 DS and follow this with the first exercise of the goal-oriented program (strengthening of the calf muscles) while walking. In other words, for the duration of these 10 to 20 DS you will be walking like a lumbering elephant.
● Keep the leg you are standing on straight.
● Lift your heels off the ground until you are walking on your toes.
● Lift the advancing leg and foot 6 to 8 inches off the ground and land on the ball of the foot.

Now do the stretching exercise (#2 of the goal-oriented exercises for running, p. 86).

Walk along for about 10 DS and shake out the advancing leg at every step.

Now do the 4th goal-oriented exercise for running (strengthening the ankles, p. 87) and follow that with the 5th (stretching exercise with body bend, p. 87).

Walk a few steps further while shaking out the respective advancing leg.

Follow this with the 7th goal-oriented exercise for running: 5U to 100 DS easy running on the spot, p. 87. You do not have to remain in the exact same place while you do this; you can gradually "gain ground". All you need do is bend forward slightly and let your support leg roll by and you are already running. With this you have finished the first part (warm up). You should do these warm up exercises in the same way prior to every training session.

*Training*    **Build Up Program, Step 1, Part 2**
The performance phase lasts about 10 minutes. You are now alternating between 20 DS running and 80 DS walking at a brisk pace. Run loosely, but concentratedly and pay attention
● to your foot position (toes pointed inward)
● and to any unevenness of the path.
● Get accustomed to what is called step breathing right from the start. In step breathing, the breathing rhythm is adapted to the running pace. The faster you run, the faster

89

you breathe. When this happens, you should accentuate your exhaling. The time it takes to exhale, that is, the number of steps needed for exhaling, can never be less than the time it takes to inhale. The normal proportion is 2:4, or 1 DS to inhale, 2 DS to exhale. Inhale through the nose and exhale through the mouth, do not strain, but let the air flow out easily. With increased stress the proportion of inhaling to exhaling should amount at the most to 1:1.

*To summarize the most important points:*
- *run loosely*
- *by bending slightly forward, roll off the support leg*
- *land on the ball of the advancing foot and follow through to the heel*
- *keep your toes parallel or pointed slightly inward, never outward*
- *practice step breathing*
- *inhale through the nose, exhale through the mouth*
- *do not strain*
- *return after 5 minutes.*

*At the end of the performance phase, in other words, after the last walking pause, you should take your pulse or determine your 15-second-count. This serves as your transition criterium.*

*Resting*

**Build Up Program, Step 1, Part 3**
Cover the rest of the distance in the manner described for Part 1, which means vary the goal-oriented exercises for running in the manner described above and perform them as you walk.

The next day's training schedule takes its cue from the transition criteria.
- Did you notice any discomforts in your legs before the next training session (in other words, on the next day)?
- Or was your pulse rate on the previous training day within the training effective range at the end of the last walking pause of the performance phase?

90

If so, the dose of the last training day represented an effectively measured stress upon your heart or your legs or on both.

If that is the case, continue the program in the described manner until your pulse rate no longer reaches the effective range and you are completely free of any discomforts. Only then should you attempt the next higher step in the build up program.

*Overcoming
the deadlock*

The length of time you will need to work through the 15 steps of the build up program will vary with the individual. Do not get discouraged if after an auspicious start you suddenly seem to be making no progress. The first deadlock indicates the limits of your present endurance capacity. It sometimes takes days, and occasionally even weeks, before you will overcome it, and not everyone is equally gifted in running. Practice a little patience and you will accomplish your goal for sure

- if you are healthy
- if you observe the transition criteria
- if you do not skip any of the steps
- if you train 6 times or a minimum of 4 times a week.

*By the time you have arrived at step 9, you have already acquired a considerable endurance capacity and will probably have noticed for yourself that you have undergone some internal and external physical changes. You probably feel completely different than you did before you started training.*

At this point many of my patients assure me that I have made a new person out of them. Of course I have not; they have done it themselves. I have merely shown them the way.

*See the
program
through to
Step 15*

Nevertheless, if I now recommend that you see it through to step 15 of the build up program, I have two main reasons for doing so:

1. The effect increases with the duration of the run, and the

91

more difficult part of the build up program lies in the adaptation of the support system. You have already accomplished this by the time you complete step 9. You can now reinvest a portion of the "proceeds" from the first build up steps in the next steps and thus make correspondingly quicker progress.

2. By the time you reach build up step 15 you can reduce the number of training sessions to twice a week and still remain "fit". This means a reduction of the total time expenditure and greater flexibility in scheduling your training.

After step 14 you can train wherever you wish. Even running on harder surfaces will probably not cause you any more discomfort. Still, whenever possible you should avoid asphalt or cement or concrete. You can now attempt with confidence the smaller inclines, even if they continue for some distance. However, you should observe the following points when running on uneven ground.

● Shorten the length of the stride and maintain the pace (shift to "second gear").

● Increase the breathing rate, even if you do not notice any shortness of breath (inhale at 1 or 1½ DS, exhale 1 DS)

● Do not develop any false pride. Take a walking pause if breathing becomes difficult.

## Phase III: Maintenance program

You have now reached the maintenance phase and only need 30 minutes of training 2 or 3 times a week in order to maintain your current endurance capacity. However, you should keep in mind that the time intervals between the training sessions should be kept approximately equal.

*By the time you are able to jog for 30 minutes at a time twice a week with walking pauses included, you have attained an endurance capacity that is usually sufficient to slow down your biological clock.*

This can almost be taken literally—for you can test it for yourself. The biological clock, your heart, actually "ticks" more slowly, probably by about 20 beats per minute, than it did before you started your training. This is about 25% less than it was. It can also be expressed another way: your heart is now taking considerably longer rest pauses. It is as if you were to take one day off after every three on the job. If you are mathematically inclined, you can even calculate the yield that your 20 minute investment returns every day. You will come up with 2500% to 3000%! Do you know any other honest pursuit with similarly high profit expectations?

It is my unfortunate lot to have to disappoint those of my readers who are not yet satisfied, the ambitious ones, who compare their running abilities with that of top athletes, or those who are encouraged by the experience of their own improvement. A further improvement of one's endurance capacity in general does not bring about any additional improvement in health, but it does require a lot of hard work and effort. The "pursuit" then becomes unprofitable. However, there is no way to measure an increase of enjoyment. This is why I fully understand those who wish to discover the limits of their productive capacities. This is not a medicinal, but rather a physical education problem and as such it transcends the scope of this book.

# Running on The Spot

*If you lack the appropriate exercise facilities or if you are hindered by obstacles of another sort, you can do your running training at home.*

It is much less stimulating when compared to jogging in open nature. Nevertheless, whoever simply wants to improve his or her endurance capacity and ascribes to the saying "the end justifies the means", can attain this goal by running on the spot. This method of increasing one's productivity claims the least expenditure of time. There is also another advantage: overweight does not represent so serious a contraindication here.

If you opt for this method, you would do best to start running right after you finish your basic exercise program. This way you are already warmed up. The procedure is simple:

- *You are familiar with the technique from the preprogram.*
- *Run for 6 to 8 minutes a day immediately after completing the basic program.*
- *Choose as your initial pace somewhere in the neighborhood of 40 DS a minute and*
- *increase the pace by steps of about 10 DS per minute in keeping with the already familiar transition criteria.*
- *Should you no longer reach the training effective pulse rate range at 80 DS/min., you can increase the effect by lifting the advancing leg higher off the ground.*

# 7. Hiking

*Required pace: 5 mph*

To dispel any misconceptions right from the start, we are not here talking about taking a walk or a jolly Sunday stroll with our knapsacks on our backs, but rather about a "walkathon" at a speed of approximately 5 mph on even ground.

*You will need*
- *healthy legs and feet*
- *a lot of time and*
- *suitable landscape.*

If these requirements are met, this method can also improve or maintain your endurance capacity. The most important rules are:
- Set your highest priority on appropriate shoes. You would do best to choose a lightweight climbing shoe that extends above the ankles. The shoe must fit well without constricting the foot. Make sure the shoe has an inner sole and is well padded around the ankle.
- If your feet blister easily, the same rules apply here as in running.
- Powder your feet and wear light cotton socks under heavy woolen ones.

95

- The training outfit is unsuitable for hiking. Slacks, a sweater, and a wind breaker are better.
- Always wear a hat, even in the summer.
- Walk at least one hour a day at a vigorous pace and
- wherever possible choose paths with inclines. This is the only way to produce a sufficient stress on the circulatory system while walking.

Under given geographical prerequisites, walking is especially recommended as pre-running training for people who may not or may not yet run because of overweight.

# 8. Swimming

*Swimming and rowing are the two endurance sports that have the most demanding requirements.*

I usually put it this way: you have to be able to *swim* and you have to be *able* to swim. That means, you have to possess the technical prerequisites as well as the skills that make long distance swimming possible.

It is a widespread misconception to think that just remaining in the water is enough to attain a productivity increasing effect. As you already know by now, the only decisive thing is

● the stress on the circulatory system, which is induced by dynamic work
● with an intensity that leads to a certain pulse rate
● which is maintained for a minimum of 6 minutes.

*The level of the pulse rate is a reliable measure of the intensity of the stress only when it is produced exclusively and directly by the stress itself and not by other factors that are possibly only side effects of the stress.*

*Incorrect breathing leads to forced breathing*

One of several factors that can alter the pulse rate is incorrect breathing, sometimes called forced breathing.

In swimming, the breathing technique is a very critical point, especially for all breast stroke activities, because
● the body is loosely stretched out in the water, that is, it should "hover" parallel to the water surface so as not to hinder forward propulsion
● while the head, and at the very least the face, including the nose and mouth, dip into the water. This has two consequences:
● the nose and mouth have to be raised out of the water in order to inhale
● and the swimmer must exhale under water. This in turn means
● the breathing rhythm has to be strictly coordinated with the movement rhythm (stroke breathing—similar to step breathing).

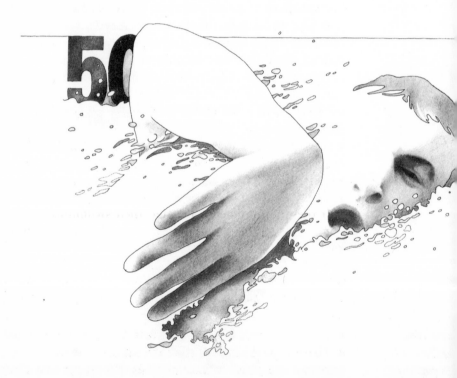

● The swimmer has to exhale against the resistance of the water, which in turn depends upon how deep the head dips below the surface. The deeper the nose and mouth go under water, the stronger the resistance. This is why you have to blow out harder when exhaling in order to overcome the resistance of the water. This is in itself a form of forced breathing.

Moreover, when the nose and mouth submerge, and when water is thus forced into the nose, a reflex action occurs whereby
● the air passages become narrower and
● a breathing delay is triggered and
● the air stream is "put under pressure" to prevent the water from entering. Therefore, when a person's head goes under water, he or she almost "automatically" experiences "faulty breathing" (dyspnea), which as a rule, is

accompanied by an acceleration of the pulse.

In my estimation, this is the more important reason why there are surely a great many people who are capable of staying afloat, but who are not really able to swim.

*To be able to swim correctly is one of the prerequisites for improving your endurance capacity through this sport.*

*The other requirement is a swimming pool with an open lane which permits continuous swimming for more than 10 minutes.*

If these requirements are met, then swimming is excellently suited to improve or maintain your endurance capacity:
● It places stress on all the major muscle groups.
● The mechanical stress on the support system is practically nil, since the weight of the body is counterbalanced by its buoyancy.

● The movement is almost exclusively of a dynamic nature.
● There is nothing better for the spine.
● Swimming offers a large number of positive side effects,

including the favorable effect of the vegetative nervous system on skin reflexes.

Of all the possible strokes, I prefer the crawl. With this, the positive features mentioned above are most pronounced. Therefore, if you want to maintain your endurance capacity by means of swimming, you should learn the crawl—from a good swimming instructor—even if you are an older person. If you cannot do the crawl and also have no desire to learn it, the backstroke is an acceptable alternative.

The next time you go swimming, you can do a few preparatory breathing exercises:
- lie flat in the water, face down
- hold on to the edge of the pool (use the ridge or the rope)
- kick your feet energetically back and forth from the hips
- with loosely stretched knees
- keeping your toes pointed slightly inward.
- At the same time and to the rhythm of the kicks, turn your head sideways, breathe in through the mouth and out under water through the mouth *and* nose.
- Take 6 breaths in intervals that are determined by the kicks: 2 beats in, 4 beats out.
- Inhale only with short breaths, not taking too much air, and let all the air escape in a relaxed way. Breathing difficulties usually derive from too much, rather than too little, air in the lungs.
- Practice diligently. Breathing and kicking must become one automatic coordinated action.

Only after your swimming form has become impeccable should you begin with the actual training program. It becomes effective when you can swim 500 meters six days a week and require no more than 10 minutes each time to do it.

# 9. Rowing

*Rowing is the second stamina increasing sport with demanding requirements. You will need:*
- *a suitable body of water*
- *a boat and*
- *as a rule a crew as well.*

This is asking for a lot. Yet, if you can meet all of these requirements, you can acquire and maintain strength and endurance. The simultaneous exertion of almost all of the major muscles immediately makes an increased demand on the body's need for oxygen and thus represents a very effective training stimulant.

*Join a rowing club*

To practice this sport, you usually have to belong to a rowing club. As a rule, you also need an instructor. He will tell you what you should or should not do, and I can thus spare myself any further comments on the subject of rowing.

## Rowing Machines

As far as stationary home rowing machines are concerned, the same applies for these "instruments of torture" as for exercise bicycles: training is nothing more than an obligatory

101

exercise and provides no enjoyment.

*There is no question that a rowing machine is a very practical piece of training equipment, yet it is only effective if it is used on a regular basis.*

Compared to treadmills, rowing machines have the advantage of engaging a larger muscle mass and thus the advantage of a lower fatigue factor. However, the stress is less easy to regulate and only experienced rowers find the proper stress level without using a device to measure the pulse. Since a home rowing machine costs considerably less than an exercise bicycle, such an investment is surely worth considering.

*Only the experienced finds the right degree of stress*

The same rules regarding intensity and duration apply for training on a rowing machine as for all of the other stamina building activities. The guidelines governing the intensity is the age-dependent training pulse rate.

*The rowing technique*

Sit on the sliding seat, resting your feet on the stretchers, which should be equipped with loops for your feet in order to facilitate the forward sliding movement of the seat. Starting position: knees bent at a 90° angle, the upper body bent forward, arms stretched straight ahead. The shoulders should also be far forward. Grip the ends of the oars from above with the thumb underneath. During the stroke, as you pull back on the oars, you simultaneously stretch your knees, straighten the upper body (without pushing it backwards), and bend the arms. The stroke is executed against the resistance of a brake located in the oarlock. This resistance, particularly at the beginning, should not be set too high and should be the same for both oarlocks. The determining factor for the level of the stress is the speed of the body movement and thus the number of strokes.

*Breathe in rhythm to the strokes*

Begin your training with a speed of 30 strokes and increase it gradually in proportion to the pulse rate. It should always remain within the training effective range. Breathe in time with the strokes, exhaling easily with the forward pull of the oars. Breathing out should last a little longer than breathing in. If at the beginning of the training the stress is too high at 30 strokes, that is, the pulse rate exceeds the level of the adjustment rate plus 10, you should loosen the oarlock brakes. A higher number of strokes is better than a high resistance.

In order to warm up more quickly, it is a good idea to work in the beginning with a somewhat higher stroke number and to fall back to the normal number of strokes after you have reached the range of the effective pulse rate. On a rowing machine, then, you thus regulate the stress in the short term only through the number of strokes and (unlike the bicycle ergometer) not via the brake resistance.

# 10. Helping You Decide

With the rowing machine I have now introduced all of the training activities which you can do to set up your own cardiac circulation training program at home. In the meantime you have become acquainted with the advantages and difficulties that the individual activities have to offer and therefore know which sport is best suited for your purposes.

*Take the test*

Nevertheless, if you are still undecided, the following *Decision Table* may help you. Answer all the questions in the horizontal columns with yes or no. If the answer is no, make an x over all the n's appearing in that column; if yes, do the same with all the y's. Ignore the empty spaces.

For example, "Do you have a healthy back?" If yes, then mark the 5 y's in the column. If you have some back ailment (problems with the spine, constant backaches, etc), cross out the n.

After you have answered all 9 questions in this way, that is, after you have crossed out all the given y's or n's, you will be able to read the recommended training activity from the vertical columns. The activity suitable for you is the one in whose vertical column all the y's and n's have been crossed out.

Should the chart reveal that you can consider two sports activities (running and cycling, for instance), choose the one you enjoy the most.

## Decision Table

y = yes
n = no

| Conditions Determining Performance | Conditioning Calisthenics | The Crawl | Rowing | Learning the Crawl | Running | Running After Losing Weight | Cycling | Rowing Machine | Exercise Bicycle |
|---|---|---|---|---|---|---|---|---|---|
| **Recommended Activities** →  | | | | | | | | | |
| Available facilities and fitness for conditioning calisthenics? | y | n | n | n | n | n | n | n | n |
| Have you mastered the crawl stroke? | | y | | n | | | | | |
| Indoor or (heated) outdoor pool available? | | y | | y | | | | | |
| Rowing facilities available? | | | y | | n | n | n | n | |
| Do you have a healthy back? | | | y | | n | y | y | y | |
| Are your legs and feet healthy? | | | | | y | y | | | |
| Are there any available running paths? | | | | | y | y | | | |
| Is your weight normal? | | | | | y | n | | | |
| Are there traffic free roads available? | | | | | | | y | | n |

# Play While You Train,
# Train While You Play

*So far I have described the programs that can help you systematically improve or maintain your productive capacity. In addition, there is a vast number of other possible ways to exercise the bodily functions that can increase your physical strength and improve your endurance.*

*Possibilities for daytime training*

These possibilities are hidden in our daily routine like Easter eggs in the garden. We will discover them only if we consciously look for them, that is, if we remember that an opportunity to do something for our body could be hidden in any activity that we either have to or want to do anyway.

We will all see different opportunities in different places. I should therefore like to list only a small selection of what are probably frequent opportunities in order to arouse your imagination and encourage you to look for them yourselves. Have you ever thought of incorporating an exercise program in your morning routine?

*Exercises in the morning*

**1. In the shower.** Do you want to wash your back? Combine this task with an exercise for the shoulder muscles. While washing, reach your right hand over your right shoulder and your left hand up from your left side and try to touch the tips of your fingers behind your back. Then reverse the procedure with the left hand over the left shoulder. You will probably have some trouble the first few times you try this.

Washing your legs. By bending your body forward and keeping your knees straight, try to reach the ankle area. If you arch your back, you will probably not be able to do it. Keep the upper body straight and bend from the hips. This will certainly stretch the thigh muscles, but is very effective.

Washing your feet. Find a place with solid footing so that you do not slip. Stand up straight and lift your knee high enough so that the thigh touches the chest. In this way you can reach and wash your foot with loosely stretched arms without any trouble.

You can repeat this exercise immediately afterwards in another context—namely, when putting on your trousers. It is important to stand up straight, because otherwise it is not effective. Hold your trousers in loosely stretched arms and climb into them from above, first with one and then with

107

the other leg. This procedure exercises both your neuromuscular coordination and your agility.

*Lift weights from a squatting position*

**2. You want to lift a heavy object.** The rule is: never lift from the small of your back. Get into a deep squatting position, keep your upper body straight and stiffen your back. You can now grasp the object with loosely outstretched arms. Tighten your muscles and, holding the weight in front of you, straighten your legs. Even if you are prone to lumbago, you will be able to lift a heavy object in this way without any danger.

*Training on the way to work*

**3. On the way to work** (or anywhere, for that matter), you can play "race the clock". This is beneficial in two ways: first, you save time, and second, you are performing an endurance exercise.

If you regularly ride your bicycle to work or to do the shopping, almost every one of these rides can be turned into training sessions.

*Active games in the swimming pool*

**4. You are taking the family to the swimming pool.** As usual, the pool is overcrowded and you are unable, or perhaps do not want, to do distance swimming, but the water is tempting. What could be more obvious than to combine the useful with the pleasurable and, perhaps even with the children, to play a few games in the water which will serve as exercise and be refreshing at the same time.
a) The Torpedo. Push legs off the edge of the pool with a mighty kick, stretching your body to its full length, and floating backwards. Who can float the farthest?
b) Roll forward out of the prone position. When done near the edge of the pool, this is a good pre-exercise for the somersault.
c) Float on your back and roll backwards. Pull your knees strongly toward the chin, then stretch the thigh, keeping the body and the head fully stretched. You have already turned over and can continue swimming in the prone position.
d) Practice your breathing at the edge of the pool while kicking your feet. This exercise has been described above.
e) This next exercise is amusing and the children enjoy it greatly. They will want to imitate it, and by doing so will

hardly notice that they are practicing their dive. Hold your breath and sink down until your feet touch the bottom of the pool. Push your feet hard against the floor and shoot out of the water in a slightly diagonal backward direction. Exhale strongly through the nose.

By playing these and many other similar games, you increase your confidence in the water. This is why they are especially good for children, yet they do no harm to adults, either.

*Tension exercises at your desk*

**5. You are sitting at your office desk.** Hook your forearms under the desk top and press up against it as if you wanted to lift the desk. Hold the tension for about 8 seconds—this is a good isometric exercise.

You can also do it the other way around: lay your hands flat on the desk top and try to lift yourself from the chair. You can also try to pull yourself into your chair with both arms. You must be careful with this exercise, because if you are strong the chair will break.

I hope these examples have stirred your imagination and will encourage you to look around for opportunities that permit you to add a playful exercising or training accent to your daily routine. Of course, these exercises can not replace a systematic training program and certainly not an endurance training, but they can supplement it. Moreover, they cost nothing, involve no expenditure of time, and—every little bit helps.

**6. Playing ball.** The same applies to your favorite pastimes that are played with a partner or in groups. You can make up your own rules for all of them. Table tennis, basketball, badminton, soccer, volleyball, and many others are not only a suitable way of passing time, but they can also contain training elements even for the inexperienced if you build them in.

*Running after the ball*

● Run after the ball. In table tennis, especially, running after wild balls provides more movement for the inexperienced than the actual game itself.

● Really get into the game. Play it with "all fours", as it were, with both hands and feet.

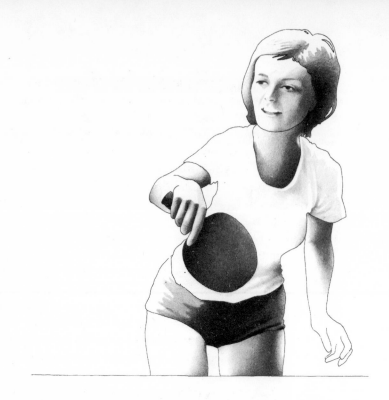

- If you are part of a team, do not stand as if nailed to the spot, but play even without the ball.
- Look upon every movement as an opportunity (for exercise) and not simply as a task.

The crucial element for the effect of an activity has always been the "how" more than the "what". If you keep this in mind, you will very soon discover that almost every activity conceals a hidden opportunity to enrich your life and make it more pleasurable. Moreover, each of these attempts will lead to an awareness of the limits of your current performance capacity and thus contribute to their expansion.

The physical productive capacity and a feeling of well-being are almost identical. Naturally they are not all there is to life, but without them there is nothing.

# 11. Basic Knowledge

*Do you
know your
body?*

*A great deal has been said in this book about the heart,
the support system, and the use of oxygen. Although we
ought to be able to assume that everyone has some
knowledge of these important body parts and functions,
daily practice shows that not very many really know that
much about their own body. And only a very few have
properly understood how everything functions together in
the wider context. In dealing with my patients, I came
to the important realization that only those people who
have an understanding of what it is all about can
correctly and enthusiastically pursue their training
program.*

*For this reason, this chapter, entitled "Basic
Knowledge", explains in an easily comprehensible form
those functions of the human body that are important
for an understanding of cardiac circulation training.*

## Muscles, Tendons, Ligaments, Joints and Bones

The skeleton is the support frame of our body. It determines

111

the body's basic form, primarily its size.

*The support structure*
The skeleton fulfills the same static function for the body that a steel frame does in a skyscraper with the addition of an equally important dynamic function. The bones of the skeleton are bound together predominantly by joints. This is the prerequisite for every movement, yet it also represents the weak spots of the skeletal system.

In order to secure these weak spots, the organism uses flexible auxiliary mechanisms which limit the free movement of the bones with respect to one another. These are called *Ligaments, guide ropes of connective tissue*
ligaments. They work in a manner similar to a guide rope, and consist of connective tissue.

From this you can already draw several very important conclusions:

● every mechanical overexertion of the *static* properties of the skeleton leads to bone injuries.

● However, every mechanical overexertion of the *dynamic* properties of the skeleton leads to injuries of the ligament structure.

Bones, joints, and ligaments together assure an optimal amount of stability and passive resilience.

*Muscles and tendons*
Active movements, however, are only possible with the help of the muscles and tendons. In this, the energy that is required for the movement is produced by the muscles and relayed by the tendons.

Since muscles affect movements of one bone against another, they necessarily affect at least two bones at a time which are connected to each other by a joint.

Every muscle, therefore, has at least two tendons and stretches over at least one joint. The tendons relay the displacement forces exerted by the muscles directly to the bones and are therefore tightly fused to them.

Tendons consist of unelastic but flexible connective tissue. They run along the flexor sides of the joints frequently in tendon sheaths, whereby the tendon and the tendon sheath together have the same effect as a flexible cable. (The hand brakes on a bicycle, for example, are constructed according to the flexible cable system).

Bones, joints, ligaments, and tendons do not in themselves initiate any movements, they are only passively involved in dynamic processes. Their metabolism is therefore sluggish, and this is why injuries to these parts of the support system heal only slowly and are very susceptible to infections.

The actually active function in every movement is performed exclusively by the muscles. These consist for the most part of muscle tissue, a fabric of cells with the specific property of actively reducing certain processes: those of the muscle fibers or of myofibrils.

*Muscle fibers or myofibrils*

Each of these fibers, all of which are approximately equal in size, can constrict itself to a definite proportion of its length and thus produce a certain strength. The strength that a whole muscle can produce depends upon the number and the arrangement of the muscle fibers that are present or simultaneously activated. Fibers in a predominantly parallel arrangement make a large production of strength possible with little constriction, whereas fibers that are arranged predominantly one behind the other make a massive constriction possible with lower production of strength. Therefore, all other things being equal, for a certain number of activated fibers the product of "strength" times "path" remains constant.

We can deduce from this that the thicker the muscle, the greater is its absolute strength, but the extent of its maximum constriction is determined by its length—a fact that is totally confirmed by our everyday experience.

In addition to their extent and their ability to constrict, the muscle fibers have still other properties (elasticity and flexibility, for example), and are able to develop different qualities regarding their ability to constrict. These qualities have to do with the speed of constriction and what is called local muscle endurance.

*Constriction speed of the muscle*

The greater the constriction speed of the muscle fibers, the greater the elasticity of a muscle. It is influenced by metabolic processes in the muscle which take place predominantly on the surface of the muscle fibers and lead to electrical phenomena which can be measured with

113

sensitive instruments in the form of action potentials.

The local muscle endurance plays a relatively large role in all types of endurance sports. Whether this quality is a property that has to be ascribed to the muscle as an organ or to the muscle fibers as the building blocks of the muscle tissue has not yet been conclusively established.

In order to understand these connections, we must realize that every dynamic activity of an organ and thus also of muscles is combined with the use of energy, and in this we see a similarity to every change of state in inanimate nature.

*Providing the muscle with energy*

The energy requirements of a working muscle adjust themselves to the magnitude of the work (strength times path) and are met through the chemical conversion of energy-rich substances with the help of oxygen, a process that is sometimes called "combustion."

Naturally, this combustion in the muscle does not involve fire and smoke; instead, it occurs with a catalytic "brake". Nevertheless, the essential features of combustion can still be found here.

The energy producing fuels for muscle metabolism are biological hydrocarbons (carbohydrates), which occur in the body as sugar and starch.

If our homes are not provided with electric or gas heat, and if we want to keep them warm during cold weather (endurance capacity), we have to store up a fuel supply for the winter. A muscle has to do this as well, especially when a continuous output is demanded of it. People store up coal or oil, the muscle stores glycogen, a form of starch.

If our fuel supply is too low and the oil dealer has excessive deliveries to make, the boiler goes out. The same applies for a muscle if its glycogen supply is too low and it is not provided with sufficient reinforcements. A muscle, however, has an additional handicap here: if something is to be burned, oxygen must be available. Now, whereas home heating has no problems in this respect, because the boiler has no trouble in taking the oxygen it needs for combustion from the air surrounding it, the oxygen that is essential for the production of energy in a muscle has to be delivered in

114

sufficient amounts similar to the way in which electricity or gas have to be delivered to our homes.

*Providing oxygen*

A muscle fiber cannot store oxygen just as we cannot store gas in our homes. This means that every muscle cell has to have its oxygen supply system, just as an apartment or house needs a gas or water supply system. And this is exactly what it has: the oxygen that is required for combustion is delivered by a system called blood vessels. Oxygen is present in the body in a loose chemical combination with hemoglobin and is transported via the blood to the very places where combustion is taking place.

Now we can also understand why a muscle bleeds so copiously after being injured; it is pervaded by a massive network of blood vessels whose finest extensions reach every single muscle cell.

The amount of oxygen that can be carried within a certain period of time to a certain place, a muscle, for example, therefore depends solely, other things being equal, upon the amount of blood that can be delivered to this place.

*Transportation through the blood vessels*

If a lot of oxygen is needed in many places of the body at the same time, the amount of blood transported has to be increased in proportion to the oxygen need. This, however, is restricted by the heart's capacity to pump blood, so that the productivity of the muscle is restricted by the capacity of the oxygen transport system and this, in turn, by the pumping activity of the heart.

*The pumping action of the heart*

If the pump fails to circulate as much blood as is needed to transport the current oxygen need within a certain period of time, then the same thing occurs as would happen if all the water faucets of a city were opened at the same time: the distribution system falls apart. In this situation a muscle can even make do with too little oxygen for a limited amount of time, just as the electricity supply can be maintained with the help of an emergency power unit or a storage battery, but this only lasts for a short time and the energy thus obtained is an expensive energy, for the muscle

*Oxygen debt*

has to take out a loan that must be repaid with interest.

115

The local muscle endurance mentioned above can be pictured in the following manner: the muscle consists of a great many muscle cells with their fibers. In an activity within the endurance realm, these cells are not all active at the same time; rather, they relieve each other like the shifts in a factory set up in such a way that the most exhausted is relieved first. This is why every muscle is capable of continuous output below a certain level of stress intensity.

*The limits of the productive capacity*

The limits of its productive capacity, however, depend upon three factors:

1. the number of fibers. The more there are available, the more capable they are of performing.
2. the extent of the glycogen supply.
3. the available oxygen and thus upon the productive capacity of the circulatory system.

# The Circulatory System

Earlier in this book I compared the human body with a state in which different groups of individuals work together according to the rules of the division of labor and of cooperation in the interests of the whole. Such a state naturally also needs supply and removal systems as well as a transportation system.

In the human body these tasks are attended to primarily by the circulatory system. The guiding principle is quite simple:

*Pipe system connected to all cells*

All materials to be transported are conveyed chemically in a water soluble form and are conducted into a pipe system to which all the cells are connected. Within the supply network a fluid is kept in circulation which contains all the building materials and fuel that the cells need.

It is as if our homes were connected to a conveyor belt system which continuously delivered without charge the complete offerings of a department store and all we had to do would be to take what we needed. At the same time we could return on the conveyor belt our rubbish as well as whatever was in need of repair or any objects that we did not need at the moment.

In the meantime, great care would be taken to see that the offerings were always complete and that our waste materials and broken parts were taken away and referred to special treatment. An almost utopian vision, no doubt—but this is what happens in the human body.

The pipe system we spoke about consists of the blood vessels (arteries, veins, and capillaries), the fluid is the blood, and the pump that keeps the fluid moving is the heart.

Naturally all of the individual parts of the system have not only different names, but also totally different tasks and are differently constructed.

# The Arteries

The arteries lead the blood away from the heart (the pump) and toward the organs. There are two basic kinds of arteries:
● the elastic type
● the muscular type.

The arteries of the elastic type, primarily the aorta, fulfill, besides the task of transporting the blood, the additional function of a pressure reservoir.

The heart does not discharge the blood continuously like a centrifugal pump, but in pulsating amounts as if from a bellows.

As far as energy is concerned, this would have injurious consequences for the movement of the blood (hemodynamics) if there were not systems available that
would tone down the "spurts" of the blood stream and transform them into an (almost) uniform current.

Here nature applies a principle that we also know from technology as a pressure reservoir or vacuum tank. It works like the air bag of a bagpipe: air is blown in in spurts on the one side, put under pressure in the drum, and can flow out of the other side in a continuous stream.

The pressure that this exerts on the blood is what we all know as blood pressure.

The arteries of the muscular type emerge directly from the predominantly elastic arteries and have the double function of transporting and distributing the blood. As a result of a muscular layer in their wall, which gives them their name, they are able to actively constrict their lumen—their internal diameter—or expand it and thus alter the resistance that is set against the blood stream.

This can then increase or decrease the blood flow to certain parts of the body and can adjust to any need.

The sum of the resistance built up by all of the muscular arteries is called the arterial resistance and is of medical interest with high blood pressure conditions. It can be measured with appropriate instruments.

# Capillaries

*Connection between blood and tissue cells*

The finest extensions of the arteries merge into the capillaries which pass over each individual cell like a net and make the material exchange between the blood and the tissue cells possible.

These capillaries are actually not vessels, because they have—almost—no wall. There is also no measurable blood pressure in them, so that the blood flows into the capillaries very slowly, and even stands still for a short time, similar to the way a bus stops to let passengers on or off. This can function only when there is more blood in the vascular area, the capillary "bed", which is formed by the capillaries, than in the delivering or removal supply network. Certain organs that are rich in blood and thus have a great many capillaries even serve the organism as a type of blood reservoir which can be called upon whenever in emergency situations the amount of circulating blood has to be increased.

118

# The Veins

The veins are those conductors that take the blood from the organs and return it to the heart. Their walls are essentially thinner than those of the arteries, for the blood flows almost without any pressure in the veins and therefore also much more slowly.

*Inferior and superior vena cava*

The veins unite to form two major branches, the so-called vena cava, one of which, the precava or superior vena cava, collects the blood of the upper body region and the other of which, the postcava or the inferior vena cava, collects the blood from the lower body region. Both flow into the right auricle of the heart.

# The Heart

The heart is a four chambered hollow muscle about the size of a man's fist and lies in the thorax (chest) surrounded by the lungs a little left of center behind the breastbone.

To the medical layman, its anatomical construction seems at first confusing. It becomes easier to understand if we think of its function as twin pumps that are connected to one another.

*A double pump*

We are actually dealing with two mechanically independent parts which have merely grown together into one organ.

This is why physicians speak of the right heart and mean that half that lies more forward and toward the right—the pump for the small or pulmonary circulation—or of the left heart and mean the other half that lies more toward the left and behind, the pump for the large or coronary circulation.

This separation is connected to the fact that, as already mentioned above, the body cells are unable to store up oxygen. Thus it has to be supplied by the blood at all times and in sufficient amounts. The transportation of oxygen is the most important function of the blood. For this reason,

119

all the blood has to be loaded with oxygen before it is pumped into the rest of the body.

This takes place in the lungs, the capillaries of which make possible the exchange of gases between the air in the lung's air cells and the blood. Nature has established an independent circulatory system precisely for this purpose, which naturally needs its own pump, the so-called right heart.

*Anatomy of the heart*

Both parts of the heart are the same size (at least as far as the volume of their cavities is concerned) and have an almost identical construction, but the strength of their walls differs.

Both parts of the heart have
● connections for the inflow of venous blood (the right side has three, the left has four) into the
● auricles.
● a large admission valve (low pressure valve), the so-called venous valve apparatus.
● the pressure producing muscular chamber and
● a small exit valve (high pressure valve, flap) as well as
● the vessel connections for the outflow of the arterial blood.

As a blood pump, the heart works according to a principle that does not exist in the same form in the world of technology, but whose action can be compared to that of a piston pump.

In keeping with this analogy, the fluid is pushed on in portions by the action of the piston and the direction of the flow is determined by the arrangement of the valves. The volume of the chamber and the piston stroke determine the size of the quantity of fluid transported by every stroke (this is called stroke volume or systolic discharge of the heart).

The performance of the blood pump called "heart" is that amount of blood that is transported within a certain period of time. We speak either of amperage (intensity of current) measured in $cm^3$ per second) or of cardiac output (measured in $cm^3$ per minute).

*Cardiac output*

This cardiac output can vary within wide ranges. At rest

120

it lies somewhere around 10½ pints a minute and can be increased to more than 42 pints per minute under a strong physical stress on athletes' hearts.

In an increase of the delivery output, the stroke volume and the frequency of the strokes are either increased together or the heart beats alone are increased. This second possibility is characteristic of trained hearts. They work economically according to the principle of frequency minimization*. The number of heart beats per minute can be easily measured as the pulse rate; the stroke volume, on the other hand, can only be measured by applied methods.

*Heart capacity of 0.1 horse power*

As a pump with a capacity of 0.1 horsepower, the heart performs astonishing feats. A 10½-pint cardiac output when at rest corresponds to the filling of a heating oil tank with a capacity of 10½ cubic yards in one day or the filling of a swimming pool 150 feet by 75 feet in about one year.

Such a small organ that can do all of this is understandably very susceptible to disturbances in the blood supply of its own musculature, to which building materials, fuel and oxygen must constantly be supplied. Unlike the

*The cardiac muscle is uninterrupt- edly active*

other muscles, the cardiac muscle is uninterruptedly active. Right from the very first day of life it performs this miracle day and night without pausing, without one single minute of "vacation". Its provisioning is insured by the blood vessels that derive from the aorta immediately after its exit from the heart and flow into the right auricle on the venous side next to the superior and inferior vena cavas.

These vessels have been named after their position and are called coronary vessels. They are the heart's most critical part and thus that of the whole organism.
● Unlike the second "critical" organ, the brain, each half of the heart is supplied by only one vessel branch.
● The coronary arteries are relatively long vessels with narrow interior diameters. Changes in the inner wall of these small arteries—sometimes called "calcifications"—

---

* transporting a certain volume in a certain time period with the least possible number of heart beats.

121

therefore necessarily lead very quickly to obstructions in the blood supply to the cardiac muscle. These in turn cause a heart attack, the atrophying of a part of the muscle as a result of an insufficient blood supply.

The loss of a small part of the cardiac musculature in itself would not represent such a great misfortune. A little more or less is actually not the important thing. But, an incident of this sort triggers a kind of panic in the heart itself and in the whole organism—which is not surprising, considering the organ's importance—which, like any panic, actually turns the misfortune into a catastrophe.

*Coronary*
*arteriosclero-*
*sis—worst*
*plague of*
*mankind*

Calcification of the coronary arteries, or more precisely coronary arteriosclerosis, is the worst plague so far in the history of humanity. Almost every second person in highly developed industrial countries dies from it, and this number is not only constantly increasing, but is also constantly including younger generations. Fifty years ago it was an almost unknown disease.

Three groups of factors have been recognized as the causes of this ailment:
● hereditary factors
● certain so-called "pre-disposing" illnesses, such as high blood pressure, diabetes, and overweight
● certain life habits and environmental influences. These include among others stress situations, a high consumption of cigarettes, poor nutrition, lack of exercise.

And with that we have come full circle. The lack of exercise is probably not in itself or as such a determining factor, but rather it encourages the development and the course of high blood pressure, diabetes and overweight on the one hand, and leads, on the other, to lazy hearts with diminished productive capacities.

Now, a heart that was capable of only slight productivity would also not be a misfortune in itself if you do not demand any performance from your body—and what "lazybones" does? But, if the cardiac muscle becomes weaker and languishes, the supply structures, and primarily the blood vessels, atrophy at the same time, and do so in

*If the heart*
*languishes*
*. . .*

122

the most critical part of the whole organism.

But you now know how you can improve the productive capacity of your heart or its blood supply and thus how you can strengthen your "weak spot".

It would surely be an error to think that training can completely prevent a heart attack. Yet, training can certainly reduce the risk, and it is just as certain that a strong heart can more easily afford such an event—should it occur—than a weak one can.

# CALENDAR

Keep a record of your progress for the first three months. Use this chart to enter the days you did your cardiac circulatory training and the basic calisthenics.

**1.**

| Day | Training | Calisthenics | Remarks |
|---|---|---|---|
| Saturday | | | |
| Sunday | | | |
| Monday | | | |
| Tuesday | | | |
| Wednesday | | | |
| Thursday | | | |
| Friday | | | |
| Saturday | | | |
| Sunday | | | |
| Monday | | | |
| Tuesday | | | |
| Wednesday | | | |
| Thursday | | | |
| Friday | | | |
| Saturday | | | |
| Sunday | | | |
| Monday | | | |
| Tuesday | | | |
| Wednesday | | | |
| Thursday | | | |
| Friday | | | |
| Saturday | | | |
| Sunday | | | |
| Monday | | | |
| Tuesday | | | |
| Wednesday | | | |
| Thursday | | | |
| Friday | | | |
| Saturday | | | |
| Sunday | | | |
| Monday | | | |

# CALENDAR

Keep a record of your progress for the first three months.
Use this chart to enter the days you did your cardiac
circulatory training and the basic calisthenics.

**2.**

| Day | Training | Calisthenics | Remarks |
|-----|----------|--------------|---------|
| Saturday | | | |
| Sunday | | | |
| Monday | | | |
| Tuesday | | | |
| Wednesday | | | |
| Thursday | | | |
| Friday | | | |
| Saturday | | | |
| Sunday | | | |
| Monday | | | |
| Tuesday | | | |
| Wednesday | | | |
| Thursday | | | |
| Friday | | | |
| Saturday | | | |
| Sunday | | | |
| Monday | | | |
| Tuesday | | | |
| Wednesday | | | |
| Thursday | | | |
| Friday | | | |
| Saturday | | | |
| Sunday | | | |
| Monday | | | |
| Tuesday | | | |
| Wednesday | | | |
| Thursday | | | |
| Friday | | | |
| Saturday | | | |
| Sunday | | | |
| Monday | | | |

# CALENDAR

Keep a record of your progress for the first three months. Use this chart to enter the days you did your cardiac circulatory training and the basic calisthenics.

**3.**

| Day | Training | Calisthenics | Remarks |
|-----|----------|--------------|---------|
| Saturday | | | |
| Sunday | | | |
| Monday | | | |
| Tuesday | | | |
| Wednesday | | | |
| Thursday | | | |
| Friday | | | |
| Saturday | | | |
| Sunday | | | |
| Monday | | | |
| Tuesday | | | |
| Wednesday | | | |
| Thursday | | | |
| Friday | | | |
| Saturday | | | |
| Sunday | | | |
| Monday | | | |
| Tuesday | | | |
| Wednesday | | | |
| Thursday | | | |
| Friday | | | |
| Saturday | | | |
| Sunday | | | |
| Monday | | | |
| Tuesday | | | |
| Wednesday | | | |
| Thursday | | | |
| Friday | | | |
| Saturday | | | |
| Sunday | | | |
| Monday | | | |